.

After Mindfulness

After Mindfulness

New Perspectives on Psychology and Meditation

Edited by

Manu Bazzano
University of Roehampton, UK

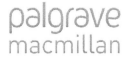

First published 2014 by
PALGRAVE MACMILLAN

Palgrave Macmillan in the UK is an imprint of Macmillan Publishers Limited,
registered in England, company number 785998, of Houndmills, Basingstoke,
Hampshire RG21 6XS.

Palgrave Macmillan in the US is a division of St Martin's Press LLC,
175 Fifth Avenue, New York, NY 10010.

Palgrave Macmillan is the global academic imprint of the above companies
and has companies and representatives throughout the world.

Palgrave® and Macmillan® are registered trademarks in the United States,
the United Kingdom, Europe and other countries.

ISBN 978–1–137–37039–6

This book is printed on paper suitable for recycling and made from fully
managed and sustained forest sources. Logging, pulping and manufacturing
processes are expected to conform to the environmental regulations of the
country of origin.

A catalogue record for this book is available from the British Library.

A catalog record for this book is available from the Library of Congress.

Contents

Tables

Preface

"Mindfulness is not a technique, but the cultivation of a sensibility." These words, spoken by Stephen Batchelor during a talk in 2012 at the annual seven-day Zen retreat he facilitates with Martine Batchelor in Devon, UK, provided the initial spark for the book you are reading.

A silent Zen retreat 'gathers the mind' (*sesshin*, in Japanese). A gathered mind is a receptive mind. I find the combination of intensive sitting and walking meditation, of working on a *koan*—all the while sustained by a temporary community of supportive practitioners—effective in fostering greater receptivity, deepening my practice, and gaining fresh insight into the way I live and work. On that particular day, these auspicious conditions helped bring forth the idea of this book.

Several eminent practitioners in the fields of both meditation and psychology subsequently accepted my invitation, contributing diverse and thought-provoking essays, which are found in this collection. If I believed in *karma* and reincarnation, as some Buddhists do, I would have said that finding such an enthusiastic response was due to the merit I accumulated in past lives. Given my preference for light-footed skepticism in such matters, I will simply say that I have been lucky *beyond belief*.

The book is a collection of unpublished essays by leading exponents of contemporary Buddhism, esteemed psychotherapists, and writers. Focusing on various practices of 'mindfulness' especially within mental health settings, it aims to bring critical evaluation, as well as appreciation, of mindfulness. Unlike most books on the topic, it offers a way forward out of what many practitioners begin to perceive as an impasse. The sheer diversity and depth of expertise assembled in the book also contributes to widening the standard presentation of mindfulness, bringing, for the first time, new perspectives.

We are in a phase of transition in the integration of Eastern contemplative practices and Western psychology. In many ways, this book reflects this transition. The reader will find here in-depth explorations of diverse approaches—from the teachings of the Buddha to contemporary psychoanalysis, from phenomenology to relational and sexual therapy, from cognitive–behavioural therapy to secular Buddhism, from religious Buddhism to mundane Buddhism, from existential psychotherapy to other-centred therapy. In spite of such wide diversity, contributors agree on the need for a greater contextualisation of mindfulness, and a more contemporary and wide-ranging articulation of the dharma.

Mindfulness programmes have so far mostly relied on a cognitive–behavioural framework, which has been influential in mental health culture during the last three decades. There are signs, however, of a paradigm shift (Bazzano, 2013). Contemporary interdisciplinary studies in developmental psychology, child psychiatry, and developmental neuroscience (Ryan, 2007; Panksepp, 2008; Leckman and March, 2011; Schore, 2012) are currently reframing John Bowlby's (2006) attachment theory into an arguably truer context, insisting that the crucial aspects of *motivation, emotion,* and *self-regulation,* present in Bowlby's original formulation, had been ignored at the time of its inception because of a cultural climate dominated by behaviourism and cognitive psychology.

In other words, we might be effectively reaching the end of the *cognitive turn.* This is by no means a uniformly consistent phenomenon, yet its varied manifestations converge. Thinkers inspired by Barthes, Derrida, and Deleuze (Massumi, 1995; Ticineto Clough and Alley, 2007; Gregg and Seigworth, 2010) have written about the *affective turn,* emphasising the unpredictable, event-like and self-organising nature of the affects, as well as the fact that they cannot wholly be translated into cognition or representation. Rather than strengthening the ego-self, the affects are a crucial expression of the embodied life of the organism.

It's early days, but if what is now limited to the world of research gathers momentum, it will begin to have an impact on how we understand and implement meditation. For instance, it may no longer be understood as a set of skills aimed at controlling the 'disorderly' nature of the affects, the chaos produced by powerful emotions, or as a tool-box of corrective procedures. It may come to mean *being with,* valuing the complexities and uncertainties inherent in being human—appreciating one's life, as Maezumi Roshi was fond of saying (Maezumi, 2001), rather than chastising it.

Many agree that mindfulness programmes have been beneficial in the mental health field. At the same time, there is a growing recognition that two crucial components have been missing so far: (1) the background (historical, religious, and anthropological, as well as mythical) upon which the teaching of mindfulness rests; and (2) the social, familial, and philosophical context in which the individual is embedded. The book addresses these two distinctive points. In Part I, 'Mindfulness in Context', four contemporary Buddhist teachers provide four different views on the background of mindfulness. John Peacock,

Caroline Brazier, Stephen Batchelor, and David Brazier eloquently artic- ulate this point from diverse perspectives. My own chapter concludes Part I, linking the broader context discussed thus far to some of the specificities present in the second half of the book. Part II, 'Beyond Per- sonal Liberation', looks at some of the societal and clinical applications of mindfulness. It calls for an embodied and psychologically informed awareness of *dukkha* (a key term in the teachings of the Buddha, indi- cating the transient nature of life), beyond the confines of a 'good life' pursued by an allegedly separate individual. This crucial point is addressed by Meg Barker, a keen advocate of 'social mindfulness' and a writer alert to the need to extend mindfulness to issues of gender, sexu- ality, and relationships. In order to be relevant, a truly secular approach to mindfulness also needs to be informed by contemporary develop- ments in critical thought. Both Alex Gooch and Jeff Harrison encourage us to consider a wider philosophical framework, inviting us to appreci- ate post-modern secularism and Merleau-Ponty's phenomenology. In a similar vein, Rebecca Greenslade traces the origins of contemporary phe- nomenology to the ancient sceptical school of the Greek philosopher Pyrrho, drawing important parallels for today's practitioners.

Within cognitive science and behaviourism there is a growing recog- nition of the need for a more holistic approach. Mindfulness facilitators themselves recognise how crucial it is to link meditative technique to a cultural, social, and anthropological context. This point is imagina- tively developed by Dheeresh Turnbull, a cognitive–behavioural thera- pist and Zen monk. He integrates the cognitive–behavioural tool-box with a Buddhist meta-perspective, the chief aim of which is liberation. Psychoanalyst Monica Lanyado provides a moving account of her work with a young patient. She offers what is possibly the most vital reminder of how meditation can aid clinical work: it cultivates the therapist's pres- ence, fostering a state of mind that helps facilitate therapeutic change.

Manu Bazzano

References

Batchelor, S. (2012) 'A Secular Buddhist', available at: http://gaiahouse.co.uk/wp-content/uploads/Stephen-Batchelor-A-Secular-Buddhist.pdf (accessed 29 May 2013).

Bazzano, M. (2013) 'Back to the Future: From Behaviourism and Cognitive Psychology to Motivation and Emotion', *Self & Society Journal of Humanistic Psychology*, 40(2), 32–5.

Bowlby, J. (2006) *A Secure Base* (London and New York: Continuum)

Gregg, M. and Seigworth, G. J. (2010) *The Affect Theory Reader* (Durham, NC: Duke University Press).

Leckman, J.F. and March, J.S. (2011) 'Developmental Neuroscience Comes of Age', *Journal of Child Psychology and Psychiatry*, 52(4), 333–8.

Maezumi, T. (2001) *Appreciate your Life: the Essence of Zen Practice* (Boston, MA: Shambala).

Massumi, B. (1995) 'The Autonomy of Affect', *Cultural Critique*, 31, 83–110

Panksepp, J. (2008) 'The Power of the Word May Reside in the Power of Affect', *Integrative Psychological and Behavioral Science*, 42, 47–55.

Ryan, R.M. (2007) 'A New Look and Approach for Two Re-emerging Fields', *Motivation and Emotion*, 31, 1–3.

Schore, A. N. (2012), *The Science of the Art of Psychotherapy* (New York: Norton).

Ticineto Clough, P. and Alley, J. (2007) *The Affective Turn* (Durham, NC: Duke University Press).

Acknowledgements

Thanks to Nicola Jones at Palgrave McMillan for her encouragement and suggestions, to Jayne MacArthur for her painstaking editorial work, and to Sarita Doveton for amendments to the text and overall support. Thanks to all contributors for their enthusiastic response and very valuable input. I thank my teachers, past and present; students at Roehampton University and the Mary Ward Centre; and my clients, from all of whom I continue to learn. May our genuine efforts and sincere practice benefit all beings.

Contributors

Meg Barker is a senior lecturer in psychology at the Open University and an existential/mindful therapist working in sex and relationship counselling. She has published co-edited collections on non-monogamies and sadomasochism with Darren Langdridge, and they also co-edit the journal *Psychology and Sexuality* with Taylor and Francis. Her research on sexualities and relationships has been published in several journals and books, and has recently culminated in a popular book called *Rewriting the Rules* (2013).

Stephen Batchelor is a former monk in the Tibetan and Zen traditions. He teaches Buddhist philosophy and meditation worldwide. He is the author of many books, including *Buddhism without Beliefs* (1997), *Living with the Devil* (2005), and *Confession of a Buddhist Atheist* (2010).

Manu Bazzano is a psychotherapist in private practice in north London, a psychology lecturer at Roehampton University, and a philosophy tutor at the Mary Ward Centre, Bloomsbury. His books include *Spectre of the Stranger: Towards a Phenomenology of Hospitality* (2012) and *Buddha is Dead: Nietzsche and the Dawn of European Zen* (2006). He edited *Hazy Moon Zen Review* and the best-selling *Zen Poems and Haiku for Lovers* (2002). A Zen practitioner for many years, he was ordained as a monk in the Soto and Rinzai traditions. He is a regular contributor to *Therapy Today*, *Self & Society*, *Dharma*, *Journal of Existential Analysis*, *PCEP*, and *Adlerian Year Book*.

Caroline Brazier is a Buddhist author, psychotherapist, and teacher, and the course leader at Tariki Trust, UK. She is the author of several books, including *Buddhist Psychology* (2003) and *Acorns Among the Grass: Adventures in Eco-therapy* (2011).

David Brazier is a Buddhist author, psychotherapist, and teacher, and author of many books, including *Zen Therapy: A Buddhist Approach to Psychotheraphy* (2012) and *Love and its Disappointments: The Meaning of Life, Therapy and Art* (2009).

Alex Gooch is a teacher, writer, and meditation practitioner. Some of his articles have appeared in *Tricycle, The Buddhist Review*.

Rebecca Greenslade works as an existential psychotherapist in London. She studies and practices Zen meditation.

Jeff Harrison is a writer, a psychotherapist with a PhD in transpersonal psychology, and a tutor at the New School of Psychotherapy and Counselling.

Monica Lanyado is a Child and Adolescent Psychotherapist. She is a British Association of Psychotherapists training supervisor, author of *The Presence of the Therapist* (2004), and a co-editor and contributor to *The Hand book of Child and Adolescent Psychotherapy: Psychoanalytic Approaches* (2009), *A Question of Technique* (2006), *Through Assessment to Consultation* (2009), and *Winnicott's Children* (2012).

John Peacock trained in the Tibetan Gelugpa tradition and subsequently studied Theravada Buddhism in Sri Lanka. He is Associate Director of the Oxford Mindfulness Centre and teaches Buddhist psychology on the mindfulness-based cognitive therapy masters course at Oxford University. He is the author of *The Tibetan Way of Life, Death, and Rebirth: The Illustrated Guide to Tibetan Wisdom* (2009).

Dheeresh Turnbull is a cognitive–behavioural therapist, and mindfulness programme facilitator at Priory in North London and Hove. He has been a student of meditation since the 1970s and was ordained as a Zen monk by Genpo Roshi in 2010. He is the author of *The CBT-POT: Learning to Play Your Mind* (2013).

Part I
Mindfulness in Context

1

Sati or Mindfulness? Bridging the Divide

John Peacock

Introduction

Clinically-based interventions using mindfulness in various forms appear to have integrated themselves in a significant manner into Western approaches to mental health care. Whether this is for people with recognized mental health problems, or for those who are simply using mindfulness for the enhancement of well-being, 'mindfulness' can no longer be considered esoteric and the preserve of a minority fringe engaged in a 'religious' activity. However, this integration has not come without a cost, and that cost has been the mutual suspicion that has arisen among practitioners on both side of the 'divide.' The divide mentioned is none other than that which is usually characterized as the clash between empirically-based scientific approaches and 'religion', here specifically the Buddhist 'religion.' Nonetheless, the suspicion can be seen as mutual. Not only do some engaged with the 'scientific' approach often view the Buddhist background as unnecessary, perhaps even irrelevant, those within the Buddhist fraternity have come to characterize mindfulness-based approaches as somehow 'dharma' light, something I will return to below.

What is in a Word?

The title of this chapter contrasts and refers to the two words used within what I am labeling the 'divide.' 'Mindfulness', for many, has now come to represent the most significant term used within what we can refer to as mindfulness-based approaches.[1] However, so ubiquitous has the usage of the term 'mindfulness' become that those practicing and teaching within Buddhist contexts often attempt either to find another word or coin new phrases to represent what they are engaged in. The other strategy, and the one that I have adopted in this chapter, is to revert to the word *sati*, a term derived from one of the primary textual languages of the Buddhist tradition. In contrasting these two terms, I will attempt to get a better perspective on where some of the suspicion mentioned above might originate from, and to see how much of it is well founded.

Buddhism and Mindfulness-based Approaches: A Clash of the Ancient and the Modern?

It is relatively easy to understand how some of the suspicion between the two elements engaged in 'mindfulness' is generated. *Prime facie*, it could be seen as arising from the clash between an extremely ancient tradition, viewed as religious and rooted in the Indian subcontinent and other Asian cultures, and a much more modern scientific and evidence-based approach that has its origins in the work of Jon Kabat-Zinn in the 1980s. Let us examine this claim.

The first part of this chapter will be primarily exegetical, as I feel that it is necessary to examine in some detail the general Buddhist background, and particularly the way *sati* is perceived within the early tradition. I believe that this is necessary as much of the suspicion of the Buddhist underpinnings of mindfulness-based stress reduction (MBSR) and mindfulness-based cognitive therapy (MBCT) is founded on both a lack of knowledge and a misperception of the teachings of the historical Buddha.

What we term 'Buddhism'[2] arose in India in the fifth century BCE and the Buddha, on the evidence provided by recent scholarship (Bechert and Gombrich, 1991), is reckoned to have died around 400 BCE. From its inception, the movement that the Buddha founded was directed towards social and psychological transformation. In many ways, the Buddha can be seen as the first 'psychologist' in that any profound change within the individual was to be achieved through penetrating insight into the nature of the mind and how it operated. His quest was to understand what he termed *dukkha*, often translated as 'suffering', but probably better rendered as 'dissatisfaction.' In the course of understanding the nature of *dukkha* and how it was generated, the individual gained insight into the part the mind played in generating *dukkha*. His aim was to help individuals eliminate their mental contribution to the overall state of personal dissatisfaction. The elimination of mentally generated *dukkha* did not have the naïve implication that everything in the world was now somehow magically transformed into an earthly-paradise; indeed, the world of experience, for the Buddha, was inherently unsatisfactory for a considerable number of reasons, some of which I will examine later. However, understanding how distress and dissatisfaction were created did have the implication that the individual who did so was better placed, both psychologically and ethically, to deal with life's vicissitudes.

Whilst the world (when the Buddha uses the term 'world' (*loka*), he always indicates the world of our experience) is intrinsically unsatisfactory, our emotional response to such dissatisfaction is to crave for things to be otherwise and to salve ourselves through actively pursuing our desires. As well as the desire for acquisition, this is also expressed through the desire for things to remain the same or for them to be different. The Buddha saw clearly how the inevitable *dukkha* of ordinary experience was fuelled by the psycho-pathology of desire. This psycho-pathology he termed *taṇhā*, literally 'thirst.' It is to the ever-present nature of this 'thirst' that the Buddha wished to draw our attention, and how, in the face of life's difficulties, we repeatedly turn our mind towards objects of desire.

The Buddha observed that we were caught in a vicious circularity; life was difficult, even unpleasant, and in an attempt to evade this difficulty and unpleasantness we engaged in behaviors that fuelled the very thing we were trying to avoid. To bring about change we needed, so he felt, to see clearly how we were implicated in the production of *dukkha* and how much of the *dukkha* that we experienced could be considered to be a 'self-inflicted wound.'

To affect this change required a number of strategies, and this is where *sati* enters the scene. *Sati* is the Pāli[3] word that is usually translated as 'mindfulness' and was coined by the early translators of Pāli texts in the nineteenth century. The translated term is originally derived from the context of the Gospels, a context that was obviously familiar to these early translators. *Sati* is closely related to the Sanskrit term *smṛti*, which has connotations of 'remembrance' and 'recollection' within the Brahmanical tradition of ancient India. The Sanskrit word *smṛti* was a term that was used to refer to texts that had a quasi-historical basis such as the great Indian epic poems, the *Mahābhārata* and the *Rāmāyaṇa*. Such texts were reckoned by this tradition to be 'recollected' or 'remembered.' This class of texts was important in ancient Indian society because the stories to be found within them offered templates of ethical dilemmas and their resolution—they had the dual connotation of 'recollection' in that they were 'remembered', but also that one learned from them by recollecting them.

In its Buddhist usage, the term *sati* preserves some of these connotations. What is being referred to in its Buddhist usage, however, is not primarily historical memory, although even this is, to a degree, preserved, but remembrance, recollection, or awareness occurring in the present moment. Indeed, probably one of the best ways of translating the term *sati* is not by a single word, but by a short phrase. Glenn Wallis uses the phrase "present moment-awareness" (2007: viii). Whilst I don't disagree with this, I would render *sati* as 'present moment recollection', as it captures some of the resonances of the Brahmanical Sanskrit usage. Nevertheless, it is often easy to overlook the fact that this form of recollection or remembrance also *learns*, as we shall see later, from past experience.

Sati does not wobble

So how do we now understand *sati*? *Sati* 'recollects' or 'remembers' what activity one is engaged in, in the present moment. This, as already alluded to, is different from historical recollection or remembrance, as this is a 're-collecting' or 're-membering' of the mind from states of fragmentation and into some degree of wholeness—no matter how fleeting this may be. Thus, one dimension of *sati* is that it enables the mind to retain focus and attention on an activity or an object, or as the language of the commentarial texts puts it "*sati* does not 'wobble' (*apilāpana*)." As the Buddha at the beginning of the *Satipaṭṭhāna Sutta* (*The Discourse on the Four Ways of Establishing Present Moment Recollection*) says:

> Establishing present moment-recollection right where you are, breathe in, simply aware, then breathe out, simply aware. Breathing in long, know directly *I am breathing in long*. Breathing in short, know directly *I am breathing out short* (Chalmers, 1994: 56).

These instructions are deceptively simple, but as anyone who has ever tried to engage with this meditational practice quickly discovers, the mind almost willfully refuses to stay focused for any length of time and thus we discover that our minds, seemingly, have minds of their own. *Sati* is, for the Buddha, not something that simply comes naturally, but something that we have to train (*sikkhati*) ourselves in by cultivating (*bhāvanā*) it over and over again. Whilst *sati* is a mental factor that can arise with states of consciousness it all too often remains in a nascent state. Therefore, the Buddha urges people to cultivate this factor repeatedly, which is present in all human minds.

The Buddha's language in the early Pāli texts abounds with metaphors, many of them linked to agrarian forms of life, and his language around the 'cultivation' of *sati* is no exception. Just as newly planted seeds need a great deal of attention so the cultivation of *sati* requires a diligence (*appamāda*) that marks a step away from the 'carelessness' or 'negligence' (*pamāda*) so often associated with normal forms of life. So important was his stress on 'diligence' that there is in the Buddha's final reported words an exhortation to be alert and diligent: "All constructions are evanescent—become accomplished through diligence" (Carpenter, 1992: 120).[4]

The movement into a life, which has *sati* as a guiding force, is the movement into a life in which the mind becomes aware of the conditions, moorings, and the character of its own activities. The individual is made aware that it is a totality of life activities, which are physiological, emotional, mental, rational, and non-rational. The four ways of establishing or founding mindfulness were thus centered on physiological processes, feelings, mental activities, and mental objects. Founding *sati* upon these was considered to be the direct way (*ekāyano maggo*) to attain liberation from compulsive and *taṇhā*-driven behaviors. This, so the Buddha believed, was the way for human beings to understand and take control of their lives. *Sati* is ultimately what orients human beings towards 'actuality'—the understanding of living, growing, decaying, and dying as a conditioned process, technically known as *saṅkhāra*.

Simple awareness

The Buddha thought that *sati* could only be accomplished or perfected through the gradual dropping away of destructive forms of desire. However, *sati* was only one element in a number of closely related strategies recommended by the Buddha. Close attention was to be paid, in particular, to one's ethical life because morally dubious and unethical behavior hardened into character, what the Buddha referred to as 'the shape of one's life.' The path to liberation was seen as composed of three elements: insight (*paññā*), meditation (*samādhi*), and ethics (*sīla*). Each of these three elements was seen as being deeply interrelated, with the development of the ethical dimension in one's life being crucial. Meditation and the cultivation of *sati*, so the Buddha thought, was a necessary, but not sufficient, condition for the attainment of the *desideratum* of the Buddhist path. Moreover, when we begin to examine *sati* in more detail we find that the Buddha has a highly nuanced understanding of its function and purpose.

Crucial to the functioning of *sati* is its ability to stay with what is arising in experience, no matter whether pleasant or unpleasant, without repressing or further proliferating (*papañca*) it. This is considered to be one of the most basic tasks of *sati*, and we might term it 'simple awareness.' The practice of simple awareness is considered to be foundational and consists of non-judgmental recognition and acknowledgment of what has arisen in one's psychophysical experience.

Nevertheless, there are other forms of *sati* that build on the foundation of simple awareness. One of these is an awareness that we might refer to as 'protective'; however, this must be preceded by the cultivation of simple awareness for it to be able to function.

Protective awareness

In the *Dukkhadhamma Sutta* in the *Saḷāyatanavagga* of the *Saṃyutta Nikāya*, the Buddha offers advice on how to conduct oneself in daily life:

> Suppose a man should enter a thorny forest. There would be thorns in front of him, thorns behind him, thorns to his left, thorns to his right, thorns below him, thorns above him. He would go forward mindfully, he would go back mindfully, thinking, 'May no thorn prick me!' So too, bhikkhus, whatever in the world has a pleasing and agreeable nature is called a thorn...having understood this thus as 'a thorn' one should understand restraint and non-restraint (Bodhi, 2000: 189).

Clearly, what the Buddha is referring to in this passage is the restraint and non-restraint of the senses, and it is *sati* that is intimately connected to this restraint.

In the *Kiṃsuka Sutta*, which follows the *Dukkhadhamma Sutta*, the Buddha offers a simile: A king possesses a frontier city with six gates. It is the job of the gatekeeper to keep out strangers and to admit those who are known to him. The Buddha goes on to explain that he is likening the 'city' to the body endowed with the six sense bases, with the 'gatekeeper' representing *sati*. It is the function of *sati* to 'protect' the individual from simply being pulled by the senses into unethical behavior.

In the *Saḷāyatana* section of the *Saṃyutta* we come across another simile. Suppose, the Buddha says, a man was to capture six animals—a snake, a crocodile, a bird, a dog, a jackal, and a monkey—tying each with a strong rope to a post hammered into the ground. These six animals from six different domains and feeding grounds would then begin to pull in different directions in order to return to their habitat. However, after a time these animals would become fatigued and settle down quietly together. The post in this simile represents, once again, *sati* and is meant to demonstrate that when the senses are 'tied' to the post of *sati* they cease to be pulled towards unwholesome objects.

In the *Satipaṭṭhāna* chapter of the *Saṃyutta*, the Buddha offers a further simile. Suppose, says the Buddha, that a great crowd is gathered in a marketplace to see the most beautiful girl in the land singing and dancing. A man is then ordered to carry a bowl of oil that is full to the brim between the crowd and the most beautiful girl. Behind him walks a man with an unsheathed sword ready to lop off the man's head should he spill the smallest drop of the oil. The Buddha then asks a question: "What do you think, bhikkhus, would that man stop attending to the oil and out of negligence turn his attention outwards?" (Bodhi, 2000: 170).

One could be forgiven for thinking that this is simply a rhetorical question. However, in this simile the Buddha states that 'The bowl of oil filled to the brim' is a designation for *sati* directed towards the body and, as with the previous simile, it is referring to a protective restraint of the senses. In the earlier simile, as well as this one, the individual has to be aware of every movement that they make either to avoid being pricked by the thorns or losing one's head. 'Losing one's head' works as a very good metaphor for exactly what happens when there is no *sati* guarding the sense doors.

Sati thus functions in a much more dynamic manner than the simple non-judgmental observation of experience which is vital, but, ultimately, will change very little. Simple awareness palpates experience, whilst protective awareness actively disengages individuals from potential unwholesome activity. I think it is at this point, with the introduction of a protective function being assigned to *sati*, that we begin to see a possible divergence between Buddhist understandings of *sati* and the 'mindfulness' of mindfulness-based interventions. This divergence becomes more marked with the introduction of further functions attributed to *sati*.

Introspective awareness

When *sati* functions introspectively, it helps individuals to recognize mental states, and in the case of unwholesome mental states to rid themselves of them.

In the *Sunakkhatta Sutta* of the *Majjhima Nikāya* we find an allegory for introspective awareness:

> Suppose, Sunakkhatta, a man were wounded by an arrow thickly smeared with poison...A surgeon would cut around the opening of the wound with a knife, then he would probe for the arrow

with a probe, then he would pull out the arrow and would expel the poisonous humor without leaving a trace (Ñāṇamoli and Bodhi, 1995: 259).

The Buddha goes on to explain that 'wound' is a name for the six senses, whilst the terms 'poisonous humor' and arrow indicate confusion (*avijjā*) and craving (*taṇhā*). 'Probe', however, is that which stands for *sati*. Once again, we see *sati* operating in relation to the six senses, but in this case acting as an antidote to the unskillful (*akusala*) states that have arisen within the individual rather than a guard to stop those states from arising at all.

What is crucial in the operation of both protective awareness and introspective awareness is that the individual remind him- or herself to examine their mental states regularly to discern whether they are skilful (*kusala*) or unskillful (*akusala*). In the *Milindapañha* (*The Question of King Milinda*) we find this passage:

> . . . *sati* has reminding (*apilāpana*) as its characteristic . . . When *sati* arises it examines the courses of the beneficial and unbeneficial states thus: 'These states are beneficial; these states are unbeneficial; these states are helpful; these states are unhelpful.' Then one who practices *yoga* removes the unbeneficial states and takes hold of the beneficial states; he removes the unhelpful states and takes hold of the helpful states. Thus *sati* has taking hold as a characteristic (my translation).

The function that *sati* performs here is to remind an individual of the various mental states arising, enabling her/him to recognize them and cultivate the skillful and wholesome states, whilst relinquishing the unwholesome and unskillful. This discriminative activity involves both recollection and discrimination, that is, the ability to recognize the unwholesome *as* unwholesome and to recall/recollect where these mental states have taken them in the past.

Thinking with the Heart

At first sight, the task of deliberately forming concepts appears to be outside of our usual understanding of the function of *sati*. However, the task of *sati* is not limited to purely apperceptive functions. Moreover, for *sati* to function apperceptively requires *saññā*, the faculty of perception and discrimination, to operate through wholesome conception rather than different forms of apperception.

This is a large and complex area, and I wish to confine remarks here to the development of friendliness (*mettā*) through deliberately forming concepts related to this.

Mettā is a an attitude of mind and heart, which eludes adequate translation into a Western language. It is derived from the same root *mid* as the word *mitta* (Skt. *Mitra*), 'friend.' In its concrete denotation it signifies 'growing fat' and, by extension, has the connotation of 'spreading', 'expanding.' *Mettā* is emotion of radiant, expansive friendliness towards everything that lives. The Buddha taught two methods for attaining human excellence: *satipaṭṭhāna* (settling in present moment recollection) and *mettā bhāvanā* (cultivating boundless friendliness).

Mettā bhāvanā is considered to be that which directly activates the heart to open up to others in selfless compassion. The final outcome of *satipaṭṭhāna* and *mettā bhāvanā* can be considered to be the same. The 'Right Mindfulness' (*sammā sati*) of the Buddha's Eightfold Path is Boundless Friendliness and Boundless Friendliness is *sammā sati*. The primary locus for the practice of *mettā* is to be found in the small, but important, text known as the *Sutta Nipāta*. This text describes *mettā* as a *sati* that should be practiced all the time: standing, walking, sitting, or lying down, as long as one is free from drowsiness.

For the Buddha, maintaining oneself in *sammā sati* is the same as suffusing the world with universal friendliness: *sati* is *mettā*; *mettā* is *sati*.

To engage with this practice requires 'creative imagination' and can be seen as a way of re-orienting our perceptual faculties through deliberately forming concepts of friendliness towards others and ourselves. Traditionally, this transformation has been effected by employing phrases encompassing feelings of friendliness and kindness. Initially, these phrases are extended towards one's self, and then towards other beings, eventually extending towards all beings.

Mettā appears to be a cognitive re-orientation towards the world, so that rather than perceiving the world through the habituated tendencies of avariciousness, hostility and confusion, and the psychological heirs to these three unwholesome roots, one begins to see the world through the dual lenses of kindness and friendliness.

The use of the phrases can be likened to a 'behavioral gesture' that involves the constructive imagination and a deliberate conceptual shift. *Mettā* can thus be viewed as the active dissolution of the usual division between thinking and feeling. It could be said that instead of trying to feel with the head, one thinks with the heart.

Mettā can be perceived as a dynamic friendliness towards oneself and others. As such, it is implicated in the field of interpersonal social relationships. Inescapably, through the development of *mettā*, the cultivation of *sati* is drawn into the field of social ethics.

What I have briefly outlined so far is the nuancing of the term *sati* and the way that it is understood within the early Buddhist tradition. What we can perceive is a movement from *sati* seen as a form of simple awareness that observes the arising and passing of psycho-physical phenomena and is characterized by a non-judgmental stance, to *sati* as *mettā*, and its implication within the field of ethics. It would be easy to see this movement from simple awareness to ethics as a linear progression that takes in protective awareness and introspective awareness before culminating in ethical relations. However, to do so would be to overlook the very dynamic that is embedded in the forms of *sati* that we have examined. Rather than a simple linear progression, what we can perceive is a vibrant inter-relationship between the functions of *sati* with the varying forms that we have delineated supporting each other. It is the development and expression of these four forms of *sati* in daily life that constitute, in early Buddhist terms, what can be considered as the mindful life.

MBSR and MBCT

Mindfulness-based interventions have their origins in the work of Jon Kabat-Zinn (1990) in the 1980s and his foundation of the Stress Reduction Clinic at the University of Massachusetts Medical School. In a recent article, Kabat-Zinn (2011) reflects on the early years and the founding of MBSR. Here Kabat-Zinn states that his own trajectory was fuelled by contact with traditional Buddhist approaches, namely, Korean Zen and the *vipassanā* tradition. In fact, he singles out a two-week *vipassanā* retreat in 1979 as being the origin of the MBSR program. He claims to have had a 'vision' where

> [I] saw in a flash not only a model that could be put in place, but also the long-term implications of what might happen if the basic idea was sound and could be implemented in one test environment— namely that it would spark new fields of scientific and clinical investigation, and would spread to hospitals and medical centres and clinics across the country and around the world, and provide right livelihood for thousands of practitioners... Pretty much everything I saw in that 10 seconds has come to pass (2011: 287).

His aim, it appears, would be to bring the essence of meditation practices to those never likely to visit a *vipassanā* or Zen meditation centre. Moreover, he states:

> Why not try to make meditation so commonsensical that anyone would be drawn to it? Why not develop an American vocabulary that spoke to the heart of the matter, and didn't focus on the cultural aspect of the traditions out of which the dharma emerged, however beautiful they may be, or on centuries old scholarly debates concerning fine distinctions in the *Abhidhamma* ... What better place than a hospital to make the dharma available to people in ways they might possibly understand it and be inspired by a heartfelt and practical invitation to explore whether it might not be possible to do something *for themselves* as a complement to their more traditional medical treatments, since the entire raison d'être of the dharma is to elucidate the nature of suffering and its root causes, as well as provide a practical path to liberation from suffering? All this to be undertaken, of course, without ever using the word 'dharma' (2011: 287–8).

I have quoted at length here because of the importance, not only in understanding the origins of MBSR, but also its aims and intentions. It is clear from the above that part of the motivation was to bring the ethos and practice of traditional forms of Buddhism into an arena where it could be of benefit to an audience that would clearly never approach meditation, let alone things 'Buddhist.' Kabat-Zinn's reflections are made in 2011, thirty years after the foundation of the first MBSR program at the University of Massachusetts, and his remarks appear to be, in his own words, a 'reflection' on both how MBSR emerged and its current state in the contemporary world.

Given Kabat-Zinn's approach, meditation was not only to be brought to audiences who would never come into contact with the dharma, but that one of its primary practices, that is, meditation, was to be subject to the rigorous scrutiny of empirical science in a clinical environment. Nevertheless, the starting-point of his approach, as that of the Buddhist traditions was 'suffering' (*dukkha*).

It is quite obvious that 'suffering' is not a Buddhist problem alone, but one that besets all humans at some point, no matter what race, religion, or country they might originate from. Human distress thus becomes the shared basis for MBSR and other mindfulness-based interventions, as well as the Buddhist traditions. It is worth asking the following question at this juncture: 'If the problem is a shared human problem, couldn't the solution also be found within the human condition?'

An answer to this question certainly appears to be there in Kabat-Zinn's approach, with his attempt to move Buddhist practices into a wider arena. Simply stated, we could say that 'mindfulness' or *sati* are not exclusively Buddhist, but that all humans have the ability to develop and cultivate what helps them deal with distress. Yet one of the major stumbling blocks that appeared to be there at the beginning of the development of mindfulness-based approaches and is still there at the present, is the term 'Buddhist'.

Is 'Buddhism' a religion?

'Buddhism', as surely everyone knows, is one of the world's major religious traditions. Nevertheless, although this is true, it takes little account of the historical figure of the Buddha (who, of course, wasn't a 'Buddhist') and of his understanding of the nature of the mind. It could be argued that at its inception the teaching of the Buddha—what is later referred to as the 'Buddhist tradition'—is anti-religious. The Buddha did not see himself establishing a religious tradition to rival those extant in the India of his time. When one examines the Pāli Canon one see a figure who is at odds with the religious traditions of his day. When speaking of the stumbling blocks that keep us bound to repetitive forms of behavior, what he terms 'clinging' (*upādāna*), he specifically refers to 'rites and rituals.' In the course of Buddhism's long history, it is figures other than the Buddha who introduce specifically religious elements, such as rituals and devotionalism. Nevertheless, during his lifetime he is intensely critical of the introduction of such elements and refers to them as 'attachments' and 'entrapments.' It could be argued that the Buddha sees 'religion' not as a solution to the problems of the human condition, but one of its major tribulations. 'Religious' solutions to life's problems, for the Buddha, tended to veer towards both the consolatory and the simplistic. However, both MBSR and MBCT have their roots in the 'Buddhist tradition', and highlighting that this is the case is often considered by some to be in itself both problematic and disturbing. Yet, notwithstanding the difficulty in dispelling the 'religious' aura, when we examine the Buddha's understanding of the mind we see something that looks strangely contemporary, despite the unfamiliarity of much of the language.

One of the great gains, potentially, of the interface between MBSR/MBCT and this 2.5-millennia-old tradition is the Buddha's highly nuanced and complex understanding of the nature of the mind. Rather than expecting individuals to accept his description of the mind in a 'religious' manner, that is, through faith, the Buddha proffered an invitation to 'come and have a look' (*ehi passiko*).

The kind of psychological approach recommended by the Buddha is 'introspective,' but this does not mean that it is not open to critical empirical investigation. The Buddha himself welcomed critical investigation of what he taught—certainly nothing was to be taken on the level of 'belief.' In the *Kesaputtiya Sutta*, the Buddha tells the Kālāmas not to rely on oral tradition, lineage of teaching, and rumor; he encourages them not to go by the scriptures, logical argument, or rational deliberation, or to rely the seeming proficiency of a speaker or because they might think 'This person is our guru'(Thera and Bodhi, 2011).

Here, the Buddha is clearly dismissing the appeal to the kinds of authority that are often sought by those within religious traditions. There was only *one* form of authority that the Buddha appealed to and that was the 'authority' of the practitioner's own experience. The Buddha believed that after initial investigation and the discovery of something of value the practitioner would then have a basis, or foundation, for further investigation. This understanding grounded in experience the Buddha termed *saddhā*, which is often translated as 'faith', but means something more akin to 'confidence' or 'trust.' However, unlike the 'faith' that is applauded in theistic traditions this is a 'trust' or 'confidence' not in mere propositions, but in one's own experience. I may be a little naïve here, but I don't find this too far from the way that scientific understanding might progress.

Methodology

Knowledge or understanding may progress, as Karl Popper (1959) suggests, through a series of 'conjectures and refutations' without there being any hope of us arriving at any form of absolute certainty. I would contend that the Buddha's methodology is not so far removed from this practice and also what Kabat-Zinn was suggesting in the 1980s. In both cases, there was an invitation to engage with a practice and to see what happens, and, again in both cases, to see whether this had any effect on the alleviation of distress or suffering. Both the Buddha and Kabat-Zinn suggest that we can turn ourselves into our own 'laboratories' in order to investigate what we find in our minds. This laboratory experiment is what we term 'meditation,' or, more correctly, 'cultivation' (*bhāvanā*) The crucial difference, however, between the Buddha's cultural context and our own is that we can now investigate what is going on, when one undertakes these practices, not just from an 'introspective' viewpoint, but from a scientific perspective that utilizes the full panoply of modern scientific methodology.

In many ways this can be seen as a plus point from the Buddhist perspective. For now not only do we have our 'introspective' evidence for a practice working, but we also have an external correlation as to 'why' these practices work, or what effect they may have on brain functioning via neuro-scientific data, and other forms of investigation.

At the beginning of this chapter I referred to a climate of mutual suspicion existing between some elements of the dharma and scientific communities engaged in attempting to understand the nature of the mind and its processes. Yet, this suspicion can increasingly be seen to be ill-founded when we examine some of the shared dimensions in relation to the nature of mental distress and its alleviation.

Let us return to the Buddhist perspective for a moment. The Buddha's teaching is aimed at the eradication of self-inflicted *dukkha* from individual's lives and the attainment of what he terms *nibbāna* (*nirvāṇa* in Sanskrit, a word that has entered the English language, albeit in misunderstood form). *Nibbāna* can be seen not as the attainment of a quasi 'mystical' state, but the quelling of behavior patterns based on greed, aversion, and confusion. The Buddha refers to these three powerful forces as 'three fires' (Gombrich, 2009). *Nibbāna* is considered to be the 'going out' or extinguishing of these fires that determine so much of human behavior in ordinary life. Glenn Wallis (2007) refers to *nibbāna* as the ability to 'unbind' from patterns of destructive behavior and, rather than likening it to the attainment of a state of being, sees it as a skill that practitioners can become increasingly better at the more that they engage with the path. This is persuasive and fits in with the tenor of much of the Buddha's teaching, which *prime facie* is directed towards the development of skills within life, rather than engaged with the kind of philosophical and ontological speculation that dominated his milieu.

It is partly, I believe, the ontological bias of the majority of religious traditions that accounts for the critical stance of many within the scientific community. After all, it could be argued, religion informs people about what exists and then it becomes the task of the individual to move towards believing this in an act of 'faith.' This may be a fairly crude representation of many religious stances, but certainly one that is not difficult to locate among those that practice within some religious traditions.

However, this is crucially *not* the stance of the historical Buddha. His primary concern is with the practical issue of the elimination and mitigation of the forms of *dukkha* that we are directly implicated in. Moreover, he didn't feel that the notion of an appeal through 'faith' to a God (in Indian culture more likely to be *gods*) was going to have any effect on the lessening of *dukkha*. In the *Tevijja Sutta* of the *Dīgha Nikāya* he jokingly likens the adherent seeking for God as someone who believes himself to be in love with the most beautiful girl in the world. However, when questioned about her name or where she lives, her parents, and many other similar questions, the ardent lover cannot answer a single one of them. The Buddha's wry comment here is 'Doesn't that man turn out to be rather stupid?' Clearly, the Buddha is no fan of theism, no matter how interpreted.

The Buddha's concern is practically based and intensely focused on the issue of *dukkha* and its psychological wellsprings. As such, the teachings he gives over the course of his forty-five year teaching career are practically oriented and aimed at the development of a range of skills that help the individual to progressively 'unbind' from unskillful and unwholesome states. In addition, his stance can be seen as primarily epistemological in that it is through coming clearly to *know* the ineluctable reality of impermanence (*anicca*), *dukkha*, and the lack of fixed essences (*anattā*) that change could be effected. Nevertheless, no matter how harsh the foregoing may sound, the Buddha's message was also infused with a vital message of kindness towards oneself and others, as represented by his insistence on the developmentof *mettā,* which he saw as a form of *sati*. *Mettā* alone was not going to liberate the individual, but it was an essential and crucial dimension of the path.

How important is it for teachers of mindfulness-based interventions to understand the Buddhist background?

Just how important is it for teachers of MBSR and MBCT to understand the foregoing? First, I think it is vitally important in helping to overcome some of the overt and often covert prejudice within the community of teachers of these disciplines, who, it should be stressed, are primarily, but not exclusively, scientifically trained; after all, much of the prejudice lies in 'Buddhism' being perceived as a religion, and in much of the contemporary world there is clearly an antipathy towards religion. However, in gaining a clearer understanding of the historical Buddha's teaching, current and future teachers may begin to perceive that, first and foremost, the Buddha is not espousing a 'religious' position; his teaching is psychologically and socially oriented, so much so, that even the ethics that he considers to be so vitally important to our forms of life and well-being, are psychologically based.

Second, we may pose the question: 'Is it necessary for any of those being taught MBSR/MBCT in an eight-week program to understand the origins and background of what they are being taught?' I think the answer to this is a resounding 'no', for many of the reasons that Kabat-Zinn outlined. Nevertheless, the foundational tradition background can be seen as an immense resource for those that teach MBSR and MBCT, and one that they can draw on both to enhance their own practice and teaching.

Losses and Gains

What is lost and what is gained in the interface between this ancient tradition and 'mindfulness' as a clinical practice? So far, we have examined this question primarily, but not exclusively, from a dharma perspective; however, I would like now to open it up to the other partner in this dialogue. I use the term 'dialogue' here because I believe that what we are witnessing in this coming together of two cultures is far from being a 'clash', but more like a 'dialogue' or 'conversation' that hasn't reached a conclusion yet, and, in fact, may never do so.

The innovators behind the development of MBSR (Jon Kabat-Zinn), and MBCT (Mark Williams, John Teasdale, and Zindal Segal) have shown both diligence and integrity in their attempts to bring meditation within a clinical setting. Nevertheless, it is easy to be critical and forget the enormity of the task that was before them. Mindfulness meditation within a dharma setting can be considered far 'looser' and possibly less technique-oriented than what we find within the protocols of MBSR and MBCT. Moreover, much instruction within a *vipassanā* retreat, for example, would take place through the medium of the 'private interview' where the instruction would be individually tailored to the person. Yet, if meditation practices were to be delivered in healthcare settings then that delivery would have to be configured in such a way as to be repeatable. In addition, it had to be something that could be taught to other trainers. This was the task that faced the pioneers of these new disciplines. Williams, Teasdale, and Segal took as their starting point the work of Kabat-Zinn and the eight-week course that he had developed as a way of working with those who suffered from chronic pain. Using this as the basis they added cognitive elements derived from cognitive behavioral therapy (CBT) that had been shown to be effective with depressed clients, which was their target group of people.

In developing a protocol that was not a therapy, despite the 'T' in MBCT, participants were invited to explore and to drop habitual frames of mind, termed 'autopilot.' They were also gently encouraged to move from the mode of 'doing' to the mode of 'being', a movement that many would consider to be a seismic shift as a way of relating to experience. This was particularly important as Williams, Teasdale, and Segal were working with those with depression (Williams et al., 2012). Additionally, there was encouragement to develop a 'friendlier' and 'kindlier' stance towards what was arising in both body and mind. The aim was not to change thoughts and sensations, but to cease to see them as 'enemies.' Additionally, there was encouragement to work with difficult, as well as some basic movements to bring the individual back to embodied experience. Indeed, the first week of the protocol was devoted to the 'body scan', an exercise of attention through the body aimed at engaging the client with 'felt' bodily experience occurring in real time.

It is not my aim to recount the whole of the development of MBCT, but simply to highlight some salient features that would be familiar to any practitioner of meditation within a Buddhist context. I think the sketch of MBCT offered above should have such a degree of familiarity. The mindfulness exercises being offered in the eight-week protocol, whilst not being 'Buddhist' in any overt sense, certainly appear to preserve the integrity of the original practices.

In what way can MBSR and MBCT be seen to gain from a greater understanding of the Buddhist roots of mindfulness? As will have been observed from what is outlined above, the early Buddhist tradition has developed a highly nuanced understanding of *sati*/mindfulness that builds on, but is not restricted to, the foundation of simple awareness. However, the protective and introspective functions of *sati* which are of such importance within the Buddhist understanding of *sati* are not so readily apparent within the MBSR and MBCT protocol. In addition, whilst there is an acknowledgement of the importance of *mettā* as 'kindness' and 'friendliness' throughout the eight-week program, there has yet been no introduction of a more formalized practice of *mettā*, with the *mettā* in the eight-week course remaining at a more 'implicit' level. That *mettā* has so far been excluded from the protocol at an 'explicit' level has been for sound clinical reasons. When MBCT was initially developed, the target group was those suffering from depressive relapse, and it was felt that formal use of *mettā* would possibly result in further entrenchment within depressive episodes. However, MBCT, in particular, is now being used in a far wider arena than that of depression and trialled in a large number of mental health issues, including eating disorders, health anxiety, and attention deficit hyperactivity disorder. There may, therefore, be a significant advantage in keeping the conversation open around this highly important issue as MBCT continues to be developed with different clinical groups and non-clinical groups.

As was demonstrated earlier, both MBSR and MBCT are, in a sense, 'newcomers' to the world of meditative praxis when one compares it with the foundation tradition, which has been around for approximately 2.5 millennia. That certain elements of practice are stressed within this tradition reflects both its profound understanding of the nature of the mind and its antiquity. Nevertheless, there is one area that is highly significant to Buddhist practice, and upon which the Buddha places great emphasis, that appears to be absent in MBSR and MBCT: *ethics*. The Buddha thought that it was not enough to simply meditate, but that one had also to address one's moral and ethical behavior. Both of these disciplines seem to have a significant lacuna with regard to this issue. Ethics, within the Buddhist tradition, was not seen to be an issue outside of practice, but part of the practice itself. As such, this is something that mindfulness-based applications need to address and incorporate into their conversation with the Buddhist tradition. Rather than dismissing any form of practice or understanding arising from this tradition at this juncture it would be wise, as both MBCT and MBSR develop, to sustain a reflective engagement with such practices. It would be all too easy at this fairly early stage of development, without sufficient reflective engagement, to throw out quite a number of 'babies with the bathwater.'

What of the accusation by Buddhist practitioners that mindfulness-based applications are dharma-light? If by 'dharma-light', one is referring to whether Buddhist thought and praxis is explicitly taught, then I suppose we must answer 'yes.' However, this is not the task of MBSR and MBCT. A more cogent question might therefore be 'Does MBSR and MBCT' preserve the 'spirit' of the dharma? I think to this we also have to answer 'yes.' Therefore, in what way do MBSR and MBCT preserve the spirit of the dharma?

First, both the Buddhadharma and mindfulness-based interventions are deeply concerned with the problem of human distress and suffering. Second, Buddhist meditative practices are being taken into areas and being made accessible to people who would possibly have nothing to do with more formal Buddhist practice. This resonates well with the Buddha's explicit statement that his dharma was for the 'welfare and benefit of the many.' Finally, the practices used within MBSR and MBCT have been developed with such care that they preserve the integrity of their origin within the Buddhist tradition. Far from being dharma-light, MBSR and MBCT both represent a profound and significant secularized response to human suffering in the twenty-first century. However, for both of these disciplines to continue to develop and maintain responsiveness to the plight of individuals both with and without mental health issues, it needs to keep the dialogue open with one of its important foundational traditions.

Conclusion

It would be a mistake to attempt to ultimately reduce Buddhism to a mindfulness-based intervention and vice versa. The Buddha's teaching is aimed at emancipation from greed, aversion, and delusion, and his freedom was a freedom 'from' these three 'fires', and not a freedom to simply do as one willed. Whilst mindfulness-based interventions may have a more limited scope, in that they aim at freeing the individual from specific clinical conditions that wreck human lives and fill them with much misery, this limitation of scope makes what is aimed for no less laudable than the intended aim of Buddhist practice. Whether a Buddhist practitioner or not, individuals usually begin the difficult business of changing their lives by addressing specific areas of discomfort and distress. Only once this engagement has begun does the vision of what is being engaged in begin to broaden and deepen. It may be that those who attend an eight-week program of MBSR or MBCT find their lives changed in ways that are not significantly different from the Buddhist practitioners. As with all forms of practice, it is the commitment to exploration and investigation that is vital, whether by Buddhist or non-Buddhist.

Notes

1. What I am terming mindfulness-based approaches includes mindfulness-based stress reduction (MBSR), mindfulness-based cognitive therapy (MBCT), acceptance and commitment therapy (ACT), and dialectical behavior therapy (DBT). All of these represent a position on a spectrum of approaches that use mindfulness in significant ways.
2. This is a word that I find deeply problematic in that it is a word coined by the Western academy to represent a tradition that is highly complex and, in its early form, I would argue, non-religious. The word is derived from the epithet used for the founder of the tradition, 'Buddha.' This word in itself is founded on the Pāli/Sanskrit term 'bodhi' that means to 'wake up.' Thus, the word Buddha means 'one who has woken up.' If, therefore, the Western coinage 'Buddhism' means anything at all, it signifies 'wake up-ism!'
3. Pāli is a Middle-Indo-Aryan language, related to Sanskrit, that was used to preserve the word of the Buddha. This is not what the Buddha spoke, but it

is a way of configuring some of the dialects that the historical Buddha would have spoken and probably bears a close resemblance to his speech.
4. *Dīgha Nikāya* ii 120. *Vayadhammā saṃkhāra appamādena sampādethāti.*

References

Bechert, H. and Gombrich, R. (eds) (1991) *The World of Buddhism: Buddhist Monks and Nuns in Society and Culture* (London: Thames & Hudson).
Bodhi, B. (2000) *The Connected Discourses of the Buddha* (Boston, MA: Wisdom Publications).
Carpenter, J. E. (1992) *Dīgha Nikāya* (London: Pali Text Society, Oxford University Press).
Chalmers, R. (1994) *Majjhima Nikāya* (London: Pali Text Society, Oxford University Press)
Gombrich, R. (2009) *What the Buddha Thought* (London and Oakville: Equinox).
Kabat-Zinn, J. (1990) *Full Catastrophe Living. How to Cope with Stress, Pain and Illness Using Mindfulness Meditation* (London: Piatkus Books).
Kabat-Zinn, J. (2011) 'Some Reflections on the Origins of MBSR', in Williams, W. and Kabat-Zinn, J. (eds) *Contemporary Buddhism*, 12, 281–306.
Ñāṇamoli, B. and Bodhi B. (1995) *The Middle Length Discourses of the Buddha, Bhikkhu* (Boston, MA: Wisdom Publications).
Popper, K. (1959) *The Logic of Scientific Discovery* (London: Routledge).
Thera N. and Bodhi B. (trans.) (2011) *To the Kālāmas*, available at: http://tipitaka.wikia.com/wiki/65._To_the_Kalamas (accessed 24 July 2013).
Wallis G. (2007) *Basic Teachings of the Buddha* (New York: The Modern Library).
Williams, M., Segal, Z. and Teasdale, J. (2012) *Mindfulness-Based Cognitive Therapy for Depression* (New York: Guildford Press).

2
Beyond Mindfulness: An Other-centred Paradigm

Caroline Brazier

Over the last two decades, there has been a notable growth of interest in mindfulness methods. From being the preserve of a few, mindfulness has come into mainstream popularity and established itself in Britain and elsewhere as a therapeutic method used for a variety of mental health problems and physical ailments.

In Britain, mindfulness has become one of the approaches favoured by the National Health Service in its provision for those with mental health needs. In this context, mindfulness groups have proliferated, teaching the approach to patients with a range of disorders from anxiety to depression, pain relief to addiction.

The growing interest in mindfulness practices has been linked with its developing relationship to pre-existing forms of therapeutic intervention and includes, in particular, the linkage between mindfulness practices and cognitive therapy (mindfulness-based cognitive therapy). This connection can be seen as pragmatic in as much as both cognitive behavioural therapy and mindfulness-based approaches study the minutiae of moment-by-moment experience, bringing together the thought processes that underlie behaviour and their execution in action.

At the same time, concern has been raised within some sections of the Buddhist community that the use of mindfulness practices in this way represents a shift away from the spiritual underpinnings of the teachings on which this approach is based. In particular, there has been concern that, at worst, the widespread use of mindfulness practices can reduce what is a sophisticated spiritual process to a somewhat mechanistic procedure. Of course, such critiques are based on observations of the worst examples of the introduction of the method, and there are many other examples of excellent practice in bringing together the best of meditation methodology with the latest thinking from within current Western psychology practice.

This chapter will explore some of the issues involved in integrating mindfulness-based practice into a Western psychotherapeutic context and will examine how a fuller and more doctrinally-based interpretation of this approach can enhance and deepen its impact on this important work. In particular, the chapter will look at the ways in which the concept of mindfulness can be viewed from the perspective of an other-centred approach (Brazier, 2009), an approach that has been developed on the training programme at Tariki Trust.

Mindfulness as Remembrance

While in some respects the modern usage of mindfulness methods as a therapeutic tool has developed its own rationale and modus operandi, the critique offered from a Buddhist perspective may enhance its usefulness and expand its scope to incorporate other aspects of the original teaching on which the method is based. For this reason, it is useful to look at the teaching in context and to review the sources from which it derives.

The Sanskrit word translated as 'mindfulness' is *smṛti*, with the equivalent word in Pali being *sati*. In understanding these translations, it is useful to go back to original texts and put the word into context. Without the necessary rigour, there is always a likelihood that a Western interpretation of the teaching and translation of the term will fail to deliver the same nuances and implications of the original terms. New implications are imported, and the real intent lost.

The word smṛti in the original Indian languages carries with it an implication of remembrance. Literally, the word means 'that which is remembered.' Interestingly, in the Hindu tradition the word smṛti is applied specifically to the remembrance of holy texts. Buddhist interpretations of the term smṛti vary but, as we shall see, the implication that smṛti carries associations with the sacred is also understood in Buddhism.

Commonly in the West, the association between mindfulness and present moment awareness is emphasised: "Paying attention in a particular way: on purpose, in the present moment, and non-judgmentally" (Kabat-Zinn, 1994: 4).

Such interpretations, based on the cultivation of awareness, it is argued, are broadly derived from the textual sources. The *Satipatthana Sutta*, in particular, and many other Buddhist scriptures, give detailed instruction for the development of this sort of quality of attention. They can be read as supporting an understanding of the term smṛti in the context of remembrance of the present moment and one's experiential way of being within it. This emphasis on present moment awareness, however, does not do justice to other aspects of the teachings, and the *Satipatthana Sutta*, as we will see, presents this focused awareness within a much wider frame of spiritual practice, and with an intention of developing higher spiritual states.

One of the leading proponents of mindfulness teachings in the West in recent decades has been the Vietnamese Zen teacher, Thich Nhat Hanh. Hanh was highly influential in the introduction of mindfulness methods, both in his own teaching and by influencing the secular mind-fulness movement. It was while attending a retreat led by this master that Jon Kabat-Zinn, who was to popularise mindfulness as a therapeutic tool, first encountered the subject (Kabat-Zinn, 2011).

In discussing mindfulness, Hanh frequently illustrates his talks by describing the practice of mindfully washing a teacup. In his book *The Miracle of Mindfulness* (1975), Hanh portrays three aspects of mindful-ness practice. First, he describes washing a teacup with awareness. As one lifts the cup into the warm soapy water, one becomes aware of the feeling of quality of the object. One senses the smooth hard china. One feels the shape of the handle and the curved surface of the ves-sel. One experiences the flow of the water and softness of bubbles on its surface.

This present moment awareness, however, is not the end or purpose of the practice, but rather its starting point. Hanh also brings into his description of the practice other aspects of awareness: remembrance of the potter who created the cup, and of the fact that the cup itself will one day be broken. These two remembrances, while appearing simple, do, in fact, allude to, and encapsulate, two key areas of Buddhist teaching.

In remembering the potter, we remember dependent origination. All objects, indeed all things, arise in dependence upon certain conditions. The teacup's existence arises upon the condition of its manufacture, of the person who made it, and of the clay and fire from which it was fashioned. In this way, in recalling the potter, Hanh is recalling the fact that the teacup's existence depends upon many factors that are not of itself.

At the same time, in remembering the fragility of the teacup and its ultimate demise, he is reflecting on the truth of impermanence. This is the second Buddhist insight. According to the Buddhist understand-ing, all things are without permanent existence. Rather, their presence is transient, being born of particular culminations of circumstances in which they arose.

Hanh writes: "One day, while washing a bowl, I felt that my movements were sacred and respectful as bathing a newborn Buddha... Each thought, each action in the sunlight awareness become sacred" (1988: 17).

The truth of dependent origination and that of impermanence are two sides of the same coin. This is a core teaching of Buddhism. In highlighting these two insights, Hanh is showing how the mindful washing of the cup is a reminder of the deep nature of experience. In the simplicity of bringing awareness to this action, the spiritual truth becomes apparent. So, in that moment, the teacup becomes associated with the dharma, the spiritual teaching, and, in this respect, is also equated as Buddha, the teacher. Hence, Hanh's description of washing the teacup as if a baby Buddha, while seeming poetic and perhaps a little simplistic, is, in fact, doctrinally profound.

Implicit in Hanh's teaching is a recognition of the teacup as devoid of self-existence. The teacup, in as much as it exists in the moment between its creation and its demise, is a transient, conditioned phenomenon. It is beyond our control to determine its origination or its end. As such, it is Buddha; it is Other. And in this quality of otherness it becomes a representation of the sacred.

The Foundation of Mindfulness

The most important Buddhist text on mindfulness is probably the *Satipatthana Sutta* (*Majjhima Nikāya* 10 and *Dīgha Nikāya* 22). This canonical text presents the Foundations of Mindfulness. It outlines a series of practices intended to ground practitioners in the core elements underpinning meditation practice, putting them on the route to spiritual attainment. The text is of such importance that it appears twice in the collection of Buddhist Suttas known as the Pali Canon.

Divided into four main sections, the *Sutta* first offers practices for the development of mindfulness of body (*Kaya*), then of reaction (*vedana*), the mind (*citta*), and, finally, mental content (*dharma*). We can note the number of points here that relate to the meaning ascribed to mindfulness practice.

We can note initially that, while the text is often seen to refer to the practical means whereby mindfulness can be attained through present moment awareness of such functions as breathing and stretching out of the arm, these practices occur, in fact, in the first section of the *Sutta*, and are part of a progression of teachings, leading to a complete spiritual transformation. Attention to the body senses is a first condition for opening the mind to the reality of dharma, the basic universal truth. The whole approach of the *Sutta* is to establish the foundations of spiritual breakthrough and to do this by focusing the mind in particular ways and disentangling from things which inhibit this process.

In the first section of the *Sutta*, we see the origins of Hanh's interpretation. In reflecting on the body, the practitioner develops awareness of its origination and impermanence. The monk is advised not only to bring awareness to the body in its moment-by-moment movements, but also to be aware of the origination and the passing away of the phenomenon, too. One of the aims of this practice is to enable the practitioner to achieve psychological separation from, rather than mentally clinging to, the physical body. By recognising its conditioned nature and transience, the practitioner ceases to assert ownership over his body and the world, and creates instead a relationship with them founded on clearer psychological separation.

> In this way he remains focused internally on the body in and of itself, or externally on the body in and of itself, or both internally and externally on the body in and of itself. Or he remains focused on the phenomenon of origination with regard to the body, on the phenomenon of passing away with regard to the body, or on the phenomenon of origination and passing away with regard to the body. Or his mindfulness that 'There is a body' is maintained to the extent of knowledge and remembrance. And he remains independent, unsustained by (not clinging to) anything in the world. This is how a monk remains focused on the body in and of itself (*Maha-Satipatthana Sutta* DN22; trans. Thanissaro, 2011).

It is probably useful here to note that ideas of non-attachment and separation in Buddhism do not imply psychological distancing in the sense of repression. What is intended is that the sense of identification and ownership is to be relinquished, so that the body or other phenomena are experienced more directly, without the colouration of self-interest. When a person is self-invested in the body, they may, in fact, have all manner of distorted views towards it. They may worry over symptoms, and fear that it is failing in all sorts of ways, or they may feel embarrassed and imagine that it is too fat or too tall or ageing. A person who has relinquished this level of attachment feels more able to relate to their body in a straightforward way. In this sense, they will be more embodied, aware of the here and now experiences of bodily processes and movements, and not imposing judgements and anxieties upon them. In Western terms, we could think of this as, broadly, a reduction in the level of psychological projection.

Having offered some practices for developing awareness of the body through the breath and through movement, the *Sutta* continues with sections on *vedana*, the reactive mind, on *citta*, the intentional mind, and, finally, on *dharma*, the most basic level of understanding available to the mind. The later parts of the *Satipatthana Sutta*, in the section on dharma, set out many of the core Buddhist teachings, including those on impermanence, the *skandhas*, the factors of the Enlightenment and the Four Noble Truths.

In his introduction to the *Sutta*, Thanissaro Bhikkhu (2011) suggests that, rather than offering four different areas of meditation practice, the *Satipatthana Sutta* presents, in fact, *one* practice, and, in its four sections, shows how the practitioner might achieve increasing levels of depth within their practice. In other words, in mindfulness practice, according to the *Satipatthana*, here and now awareness of the body is *the first step*, and as practice deepens, the whole Buddhist understanding of the nature of experience is revealed through the lens of that practice. The practice is one of delving into the experience, stripping away those elements that are conditioned by assumption and expectation, and allowing it to exist free from such elaboration. This raw experience, freed from the games of the unenlightened mentality, is the essence of the ultimate spiritual perspective.

Mindfulness teaching is therefore deeply embedded within the whole understanding of the Buddhist tradition. In this context, to interpret mindfulness simply as a practice of awareness in the present moment would be to overlook a large proportion of this core text.

Other-centred Theory

The other-centred approach offers a model of psychotherapy that is grounded in the Buddhist understanding of the mind and human process. Based on an appreciation of the way in which ordinary human perception is conditioned and our experience of the world distorted through our search for security, it aims to explore the roots of that conditioning and to facilitate a more direct encounter with the world as it is, free from the colouration imposed by our mental insecurity.

Buddhist psychology suggests that in response to our existential position as mortal beings—subject to sickness, old age, and loss—we tend to create a semblance of permanence by mentally clinging to the familiar. Faced with ever-changing circumstances, we try to create order out of the chaos and unpredictability of life by clinging to people and things that support our sense of identity. Technically, such people and things are referred to as 'objects', being the objects of the senses, which are the organs of attachment in the Buddhist paradigm.

In this process of clinging, we tend to view others in a functional way, using them to confirm our sense of self. The self is thus a product of the object of attention in any given moment. As a result of this process, we can say that the self is object-related. In other words, it depends upon the objects to which we give attention, and those objects are perceived through the distortion of the need for identity rather than being perceived in their own right.

Buddhist practice is primarily concerned with unhooking from this attachment to self-invested view. As we saw in the *Satipatthana Sutta*, by observing the detail of the process in as objective and unbiased a way as possible, the practitioner develops clear sight, and minimises the effect of self-building.

Other-centred therapy puts its focus primarily on the perceptual experience. By recognising that the mental structures and the world view are mutually conditioning—that because we perceive things according to our need for identity, our view is built on preconceptions, and that perception, in turn, supports the maintenance of the sense of self—the approach tends to look upon the world view aspect of this cyclical relationship as the point most amenable to modification.

We are often willing to adjust our perception of others in a way that we are not prepared to adjust our opinion of ourselves. This approach therefore explores the perceptual object in terms of its conditioned nature (*rupa*) and also explores the actual object on which the perception is founded—a thing which is real, other, and, ultimately, unknowable.

According to these principles, the rupa quality of the object is the protective shield that the self creates and maintains for its own continued existence. It masks the world, which is both raw (a place where basic existential anguish cannot be eradicated) and beautiful. Our view is contaminated by self-interest. Without the conditioning which this colouration imposes, life is experienced in a direct, clear way.

Within this methodology, therapy sometimes entails an examination of the nature of the conditioned view, with an intention of challenging or modifying it—or, alternatively, inviting the client to explore the experience of the other more directly, knowing that, inevitably, in ordinary

human circumstances, such perception can only ever be an approxima-
tion. This way of working recognises that behind the process which has
given rise to the conditioned view, there generally lie painful and fright-
ening experiences from the past, in the present, or in an anticipated
future. It is fear of this kind that prevents people from discovering their
full potential. By addressing the world view, therapy encourages a more
open engagement with life. Because the mind is invited to become less
attached to a rigidly-held view, the person begins to encounter others
more freely and directly.

Other-centred Approach and Mindfulness

In our examination of the Buddhist understanding of mindfulness we
saw how the latter can be understood not only as 'here and now awareness', but also as an engagement with the spiritual dimension and
the deeper truth, which gives rise to that 'here and now' presence.
In particular, we saw how mindfulness is remembrance. In terms of the
Satipatthana Sutta, this is remembrance of dharma, the deepest layer of
spiritual truth.

To put this in a psychological context, mindfulness is concerned with
the remembrance of the deep truth embodied in reality. As such, it
sits on the knife-edge between the psychological and spiritual. Just as
the *Satipatthana Sutta* brings together the mundane observance of bodily process with the most profound teachings of the Buddhist faith, so
too, as we engage the object world, we see in the particular things that
we encounter both mundane objects and windows into the spiritual
dimension. Another way to think about mindfulness, therefore, is as
remembrance of the sacred.

While modern psychotherapy has attempted to divorce itself from
notions of the mystical, it is impossible to truly construe a system of
thought relating to mental health that does not embrace this dimension. Our thoughts and emotions rest on the foundation of the beliefs
and values we hold. Our sense of meaning and connection to the greater
forces behind human existence inevitably forge our ordinary mentality.

To mindfully encounter another is to appreciate within that other
the greater mystery which is beyond the control of the self-making
mind. In ordinary mentality, the other is limited, distorted in order to fit
with the known. Transcending this distortion, the person who is truly
mindful would be fearless in meeting with the unknown. The other, an
unpredictable stranger, would be welcomed, not just in their own inherent beauty, but as an embodiment of the greater truth. In this encounter,

as the calculating self is abandoned, or at least restricted, the other, the focus of unencumbered relationship, becomes Buddha. In such a meeting, the other becomes the teacher and the source of awakening from the confines of self-preoccupation.

It is in our day-to-day encounters that our tendency to make assumptions and, in Western terminology, to project onto others, creates limitations and difficulties. With those to whom we are closest, we commonly direct unrealistic hopes and expectations. We tend to hold onto the past, often viewing people in the same light as we have seen them for years or even decades. We bring to new relationships the shadows of previous encounters, imposing transference and other similar phenomena. As we look at the conditioned quality of such relationships, we become more aware of these layers, of their roots in the past and in present associations, and we start to unpick the more insidious aspects of this process.

Vedana—The Second Foundation

The first foundation of mindfulness, as presented in the *Satipatthana Sutta*, is the body. The second foundation is vedana. Vedana is the reactive stage in the process of self-creation. It is the means by which the object of attention is grasped or rejected by the clinging mind. Therapeutic work in this paradigm involves challenging rupa colouration, which muddies encounters, and investigating the reality which may lie behind distorted perceptions. In this process, by noticing the reactivity associated with it, we become aware of the level of significance of the object. Vedana reveals which objects carry the heaviest rupa colouration because the more powerful the object, the stronger our reaction to it.

When a person talks about their experience, they will often give emphasis to those things that are most potent in conditioning their sense of identity. The objects that are most powerfully rupa for us are highlighted in speech by tone of voice, gesture, and other emphatic behaviour. When we perceive an object that is significantly linked to our identity, we tend to react strongly towards it. This happens through an attractive or aversive attachment. In other words, we are strongly drawn to it or we reject it. Vedana is the name given to this step in the process of conditioning. It is the immediate grasping or rejecting impulse of the mind.

Vedana is pre-verbal, a simple visceral response to the sensory engagement with the object. We see something, we want it. We hear something, we reject it. It happens before we have even recognised our associations or stories about the experience. By bringing mindfulness to this impulse, we learn to recognise the point at which the mind grasps the object. This is the point where personal investment is made in the world view. Bringing mindful awareness to vedana gives space for reactivity to dissipate rather than being acted out. Thus, by reducing the effect of our reactions, we invite a different relationship with the world. Instead of always grasping, we are more likely to perceive the objects that we encounter with respect and reverence, knowing that they exist in and of themselves, and not for our personal benefit or in order to harm us.

Mindfulness and Embodied Phenomenology

When we read the *Satipatthana Sutta*, we are presented with a methodology. This methodology relies upon dispassionate observation of phenomena. As such, it has some parallels with the Western European philosophy known as phenomenology and those therapeutic approaches that have derived from it. This movement, which has its roots in the work of Edmund Husserl (1999) in the early twentieth century, represented an attempt to transcend theory and enquiry into the nature of things by setting aside preconceptions using a process known as *epoché* or, more commonly, 'bracketing.' This phenomenological method involved increasingly fine layers of investigation, which refined the quality of perception by systematically eliminating the strata of common assumption and personal association.

Buddhist methods of spiritual development, practised through meditation, and also through mindfulness in daily life, similarly seek to set aside the attachment-building processes of attraction and aversion, and to perceive phenomena as they exist, devoid of self-contamination. The first section of the *Satipatthana Sutta* focuses on awareness of the breathing and of other aspects of bodily experience, exploring them with this kind of objectivity. Awareness is developed in the physical activity of daily life: in walking, standing, and lying down, and in functions such as eating, getting dressed, falling asleep, waking up, talking, and so on. The text suggests that this awareness be cultivated through observation of the body, "in and of itself", and "not sustained by anything in the world" (DN22.1; trans. Thanissaro, 2011).

The latter phrase is not intended to imply a disconnection in the sense of otherworldliness, but rather suggests that the body be perceived as something which is existent in itself, free of the attachments of association. A body is a body is a body. It is not self but 'other' and thus always, in some senses, a fresh experience of the unknown. In this way, the enquiry that is encouraged by the *Satipatthana Sutta* aims at objectivity. The practitioner seeks to establish a dispassionate perspective. Even the physical body is not something that we can use in order to maintain and build the defensive structure of self with which we identify. It, too, is impermanent and not under our control.

We can thus see that in the description of mindfulness of the body a practice is being offered which, on the one hand, aspires to the clarity of descriptive process that we find in phenomenology and, on the other hand, is grounded in an experiential, inner observation of the felt sense of the body state. The practice brings the attention of the practitioner to the direct bodily experience but discourages him or her from feeling personal ownership of that experience.

In psychotherapy, the therapist's embodied presence is an important foundation for the therapeutic encounter. By cultivating solid groundedness, he or she is able to offer the client stability, which persists even when chaotic feelings or thoughts are being explored. This groundedness, as described in a model developed by the Japanese Shin Buddhist psychologist Saiko (2001), can be thought of as a manifestation of faith. In Saiko's model, the meeting between therapist and client is supported by conditions that are greater than either of them. To put this in Saiko's more religious language, they are held by the universal quality of the measureless Buddha. While this support is equally available to both therapist and client, it is, however, only the therapist who recognises this fact. Only through the experience of being with the therapist in this state of trust does the client gradually discover his or her own trust and loosen their defences.

Thus, the therapist's ability to be mindful, to stay with what arises— without grasping at things that are presented in order to fit them into a personal blueprint—is itself the foundation of therapeutic change. In this respect, the therapist's own spiritual practice is fundamental to the success of the encounter. This practice, however, not only involves developing a calm presence, but also incorporates a deepening connection to the spiritual dimension—however that is conceived. The therapist's faith is important. Thus, the quality of the therapeutic relationship that the therapist offers is founded in mindfulness in two respects: in the sense of present awareness and of remembrance of the sacred.

In this foundational presence, the quality of experience offered by the therapist is not abstract but embodied. The therapist, according to Saiko's diagrammatic representation, experiences the presence of universal supportive conditions, personified as the presence of Buddha, as the base strata of the therapeutic encounter, underpinning the meeting with the client. This sense that the spiritual ground in which therapy takes place has a spatial location aligns with the bodily sense of groundedness, which can be cultivated through meditation practice or other exercises.

In both instances, the felt sense of support and the cultivated experience of embodiment suggest a primary relationship with the earth on which the practitioner, or in this case the therapist, is sitting. The contact is experienced not as a cerebral concept but as a bodily phenomenon. Mind and body unite to bring an experience that is not simply in the imagination, but rather involves the felt sense of particular muscle systems, and the process of relaxation and attentive awareness. In such awareness, the place of personal investment and interpretation gives way to a more direct and unfiltered experience of the act of sitting. The therapist, in bringing awareness of this kind to the body experience, has no room to indulge identification.

Mindfulness as a Therapeutic Spirituality

While those working in the public sector are unlikely to directly engage with the doctrinal principles that teachings on mindfulness propound in their professional context, I believe that it is still possible to bring the spirit of reverence and other-focused enquiry into mindfulness-based therapies. Indeed, given the inseparable relationships between mental health and the spiritual well-being of the person, as well as their relationship to the real material world, a spiritually grounded interpretation of the teaching may provide a significant contribution to this field. In providing a model that engages with the spiritual dimension through a deeper appreciation of the mystery of the other, this approach offers a model that is not only therapeutic, but also looks towards a secular spirituality and a response to people's deepest need for meaning and a sense of place in the universe.

The fundamental proposition of the mindfulness teachings is that by bringing attention into the action, the spiritual aspect of experience is revealed. This article of faith may, perhaps, provide a modus operandi for those practitioners and therapists who voice concern about the secularisation and appropriation of this method. If mindful awareness of phenomena as they arise will naturally lead us toward the spiritual dimension, then as mindfulness is taught, and those practising it continue to develop in sophistication and depth of connection to the method, that in itself may create the conditions for the kind of spiritual revolution that some would seek.

As an other-centred practitioner, my own orientation leads me to invest in those aspects of the method that bring about a more honest and precise relationship with the physical world, knowing that through this mundane connection to the material, a deeper spiritual connection is fostered. The facts are friendly, and mindful investigation into the nature of experience (so long as it incorporates an attitude which does not buy into the glorification of the self which is sometimes found in popular Western psychology circles) can be fruitful and liable to lead to healthier mental states.

Conclusion

The practice of mindfulness has become popular in a variety of spheres in recent years. This popularity has resulted in the growth of many courses and groups focused on the application of techniques that have been loosely, or sometimes more faithfully, derived from Buddhist sources. While these approaches are generally found to be helpful by those who participate in them, many remain primarily classes that teach methods for slowing down, relaxing, and bringing more awareness into the present moment. These methods are not at odds with the spirit of the Buddhist teachings on mindfulness, as found in the *Satipatthana Sutta* and other texts, but they may fall short of addressing the fundamental principles of the original mindfulness teachings, and they may fail to honour the aspects of mindfulness that relate to the sacred.

Mindfulness is a way of being. It is not a technique, so much as a quality of mind. As such, in its original context, it can be seen as the foundation of spiritual practice, but also as its culmination. In the therapeutic arena it offers tools that likewise may start a person on a path that can later bring increasing depth and insight. Thus, mindfulness practices offer a method that can be revisited on many levels. With the growth of mindfulness-based therapies, it is to be hoped that this reappraisal and rediscovery of the core spirit of the teaching continues.

References

Brazier, C. (2009) *Other-Centred Therapy* (Ropley: O-Books).

Hanh, N. (1975) *The Miracle of Mindfulness* (Boston, MA: Beacon Press).

Hanh, N. (1988) *The Sun My Heart* (Rocklin, CA: Parallax).

Husserl, E. (1999) *Basic Writings in Transcendental Phenomenology* (Bloomington, IN: Indiana University Press).

Kabat-Zinn, J. (1994) *Wherever You Go, There You Are: Mindfulness Meditation in Everyday Life* (New York: Hyperion).

Kabat-Zinn, J. (2011) 'Some Reflections on the Origins of MBSR', in Williams, W. and Kabat-Zinn, J. (eds) *Contemporary Buddhism*, 12, 281–306.

Saiko, G. (2001) 'Dharma-based Person-Centered Approach in Japan', paper presented at the 8th International Person-Centered Approach Forum in Japan, 2001.

Thanissaro, B. (2011) Introduction to Maha-satipatthana Sutta: The Great Frames of Reference (DN 22), translated from the Pali by Thanissaro Bhikkhu, *Access to Insight*, available at: http://www.accesstoinsight.org/tipitaka/dn/dn.22.0.than.html (accessed 6 June 2013).

3
The Everyday Sublime

Stephen Batchelor

The Experience of the Everyday Sublime

Meditation originates and culminates in the everyday sublime. I have little interest in achieving states of sustained concentration in which the
sensory richness of experience is replaced by pure introspective rapture.
I have no interest in reciting mantras, visualizing Buddhas or *mandalas*,
gaining out-of-body experiences, reading other people's thoughts, practicing lucid dreaming, channelling psychic energies through chakras,
let alone absorbing my consciousness in the transcendent perfection of
the Unconditioned. Meditation is about embracing what is happening
to this organism as it touches its environment in this moment. I do
not reject the experience of the mystical. I only reject the view that the
mystical is concealed behind what is merely apparent, that it is anything
other than what is occurring in time and space right now. The mystical
does not transcend the world, but saturates it. "It is not how things are
in the world that is mystical" noted Wittgenstein in 1961, "but that it
exists" (1961: 88).

The experience of the sublime exceeds our capacity for representation. The world is excessive: every blade of grass, every ray of sun, every
falling leaf is excessive. None of these things can be adequately cap-
tured in concepts, images, or words. They overreach us, spilling beyond
the boundaries of thought. Their sublimity brings the thinking, calculating mind to a stop, leaving one speechless, overwhelmed with either
wonder or terror. Yet for the human animal who delights and revels in
her place, who craves security, certainty, and consolation, the sublime
is banished and forgotten. As a result, life is rendered opaque and flat.
Each day is reduced to the repetition of familiar actions and events,
which are blandly comforting, but devoid of an intensity we both yearn

for and fear. We crave stimulation, we long for a temporary derangement of the senses, we seek opportunities to lose ourselves in rapture or intoxication. Yet once we have tasted such ecstasies, we often sink back with a sigh of relief into the dullness of routine.

To experience the everyday sublime one needs to dismantle piece by piece the perceptual conditioning that insists on seeing oneself and the world as essentially comfortable, permanent, solid, and mine. It means to embrace suffering and conflict, rather than to shy away from them, to cultivate the radical attention (*yonisomanasikāra*) that contemplates the tragic, changing, empty, and impersonal dimensions of life, rather than succumbing to fantasies of self-glorification or self-loathing. This takes time. It is a lifelong practice.

The everyday sublime is our ordinary life experienced from the perspective of the Four Tasks (Batchelor, 2012). At the conclusion of his first discourse, the *Turning of the Wheel of Dharma*, the Buddha declared that he could not consider himself to be fully awake until he had recognized, performed, and accomplished these four tasks, namely: (1) fully knowing *dukkha*, (2) letting go of craving, (3) experiencing the stopping of craving, and (4) creating and cultivating the eightfold path. In more idiomatic language, this means that awakening entails (1) an openhearted embrace of the totality of one's existential situation, (2) a willingness to let go of the habitual reactive patterns of thought and behavior that arise in response to that situation, (3) a conscious valorization of those moments in which you know for yourself that such reactive patterns have stilled to the point where they will no longer determine your responses to life situations, and (4) a commitment to a way of living that emerges from such stillness and encompasses every aspect of your humanity: your vision, thoughts, words, deeds, work, application, mindfulness, and concentration.

Understood in this way, meditation is not about gaining proficiency in technical procedures claimed to guarantee attainments that correspond to the dogmas of a particular religious orthodoxy. Nor is its goal to achieve a privileged, transcendent insight into the ultimate nature of reality, mind or God. In the light of the Four Tasks, meditation is the *ongoing cultivation of a sensibility*, a way of attending to every aspect of experience within a framework of ethical values.

I do not dispute that monks and yogins in Buddhist cultures have developed spiritual technologies to a high degree in the course of their history, resulting in levels of mental refinement, control and absorption that may seem incredible to modern Westerners. Yet, from a Buddhist perspective, the value of these attainments lies not in the fact that they are humanly possible, but whether they contribute to the practice of the Four Tasks. I do not find it hard to imagine how one could be highly accomplished in certain meditative techniques, yet fail to embrace whole-heartedly the condition of *dukkha* that pervades the life of oneself and others, fail to let go of the self-centered cravings that arise in response to *dukkha*, fail to experience moments when such craving stops, and fail to cultivate a radically different way of being in this world.

As a sensibility, meditation is embodied, receptive, and perplexed. It enables one to cultivate an understanding of moment-to-moment experience much as one develops an appreciation of art or poetry or nature. Grounded in the body and the senses, it values an open-mindedness to what is unfamiliar, probes one's sensorium with relentless curiosity, listens attentively to what others have to say, is willing to suspend habitual attitudes and opinions, and questions what is going on instead of simply taking things for granted. The disengagement of meditation is not an aloof regard (or disregard), but a perspective that opens up another kind of response to what is happening. And it begins with the breath, our primordial relationship to the flesh of the world in which are embedded.

Practice extends to everything we do

In the Buddha's time, it was impossible to wander through the countryside of north India during the 3 months of monsoon because the rivers flooded and the paths and roads became muddy torrents. He and his followers would settle in a park or grove, dedicating themselves to discussion and contemplation. Inevitably, people became curious as to what this man would do during these retreats. Why, they may have asked, did the 'Awakened One' have to practice meditation at all? Here is the answer Gotama told his followers to give such people:

> During the rain's residence, friend, the Teacher generally dwells in concentration through mindfulness of breathing... [For] if one could say of anything: 'this is a noble dwelling, this is a sacred dwelling, this is a *tathāgata*'s dwelling,' it is of concentration through mindfulness of breathing that one could truly say this (Bodhi, 2000: 1778).

This passage shows, I believe, how awareness grounded in the breath is the foundation of all the contemplative tasks taught by Gotama and his followers. At its core, meditation is an existential 'dwelling' within the primary rhythms of the body that link one seamlessly to the biosphere. As a discipline, it involves constant vigilance that prompts one to keep returning to the felt embodiment of experience that is so easily forgotten through getting 'eaten up' by the rush of thoughts in one's head.

In calling it a 'sacred dwelling' (*brahmavihāra*), Gotama does not hesitate to employ a term commonly used to refer to a god (*brahma*) in a non-theistic context. Here, the 'sacred' no longer denotes a supramundane deity, but refers to the everyday sublime that is revealed when the mind becomes still and focused through settling into the rhythm of one's breathing. The sacred is not found in a transcendent realm beyond oneself or the world, but is disclosed here and now once the mind relaxes, quietens, and becomes clearer and sharper as attention stabilizes on the breath. The 'sacred' dimension of experience opens up as one lets go of the constrictive, obsessive concern with 'me' and 'mine', thereby allowing a return to a world that transcends my petty interests. Such a world is excessive; it is not a manageable place. It pours forth relentlessly, voluptuously, but is gone by the time you reach out to seize it and freeze it.

In considering mindfulness of breathing as a *brahmavihāra*, Gotama places it in the company of the better-known 'sacred dwellings' of loving kindness, compassion, sympathetic joy, and equanimity. As focusing on the breath grounds oneself in the very rhythm of life, it allows one to feel the same rhythm that animates other sentient creatures and realize an empathetic rapport with all that breathes. Such openhearted equanimity provides the foundation for wishing all others to be well (loving kindness), wishing them not to suffer (compassion), and rejoicing in their good fortune (sympathetic joy). That such dwellings extend to "all beings" confirms that these wishes likewise partake of sublimity. They are not calculated desires, the fulfillment of which is judged in terms of achieving a satisfactory result, but the yearnings of a sensibility that cannot hold itself back itself any more than the sun can restrain itself from radiating light and heat. "Sentient beings are numberless", says the equally irrational Zen vow, "but I promise to liberate them all."

To practice such meditative dwelling, one needs to find a quiet place, such as a woodland or an empty chapel, sit down with a straight back beneath a tree or on a pew, and turn one's attention to what it feels like to be breathing in and out. One lets the breath arise and be released without any conscious interference. One learns to anchor one's attention in its natural rhythm, without drifting off into trains of thought or succumbing to drowsiness. Yet as soon as you become self-conscious of your breathing, the breath tends to feel forced and deliberate. You start to think of it as 'mine', rather than an impersonal process. Instead of the body just breathing in and out unprompted, which it does as long as you are *not* attending to it, the breather assumes control of the process. Now you have to relax your attention, but without losing your heightened awareness of the breath. Pretend that you are waiting, as a disinterested observer, to catch the body in the act of inhaling and exhaling of its own accord. Then, suddenly, perhaps with a shock, you will notice the breath just happening.

When asked by the intellectual monk Mahā Koṭṭhita about "freedom of mind through emptiness", the Buddha's disciple, Sāriputta, replied: "When one has gone to the forest or to the root of a tree or an empty hut, one reflects: 'All this is empty of a self or what belongs to a self.' This is the freedom of mind through emptiness" (Ñāṇamoli and Bodhi, 1995: 394). One retreats to the wilderness in order to dwell in a region that is free from human ownership and control. In the absence of anyone else to impress or flatter, one is able to recover a natural dignity based on one's awed participation in, and indebtedness to, life itself. The solitude of the natural world thus becomes a metaphor for emptiness, a sublime revelation of selflessness, an abode of freedom and ease. Such emptiness, as another *sutta* declares, is the "dwelling of a great person" (Ñāṇamoli and Bodhi, 1995: 1143).

Like the birds and deer, you do not intend to breathe in any particular way. The *sutta*s do not prescribe a right or approved way of breathing. If your breath is shallow and unsteady, then it is shallow and unsteady. You just let the body be the body, let the breathing breathe, while remaining fully aware of what is happening. As you settle into this practice, not only does the mind gradually become more focused and calm, but you notice how the experience of breathing is not limited to the nostrils, windpipe, lungs, and diaphragm, but rises and falls as a tidal rhythm throughout the entire body. "I shall breathe in experiencing the whole body; I shall breathe out experiencing the whole body. I shall breathe in and out calming the body's inclination (to breathe)" (Ñāṇamoli and Bodhi, 1995:146).

Gotama compares such a person to a skilled wood-turner, who understands the effect the slightest movement of his hands and fingers will have on the wood being worked on the lathe. This analogy illustrates how mindfulness is not just about stepping back and passively noticing what is passing before one's inner eye. It involves an exploratory and potentially transformative relationship with the pulsing, sensitive, and conscious "material" of life itself. Such radical attention heightens mindful awareness, intensifies curiosity about and investigation of what is unfolding, stimulates an energetic application to the task, induces a sense of delight in what one is doing, and leads to tranquility, concentration, and equanimity.

Nor is such meditation exclusively confined to what one does in a formal seated posture. "When walking, one understands: 'I am walking'; when standing, one understands: 'I am standing'; when lying down, one understands: 'I am lying down'" (Ñāṇamoli and Bodhi, 1995: 146). The practice extends to everything we do. To associate mindfulness primarily with sitting on a cushion for a prescribed length of time is to limit its effectiveness. The aim is to integrate mindful attention into the totality of one's conscious life. This is clear from the following passage, repeated throughout the canon, which describes how such a person behaves (I have secularized and re-gendered the terminology):

> She is one who acts with full awareness when leaving and returning, when looking ahead and looking back, when flexing and extending her limbs, when wearing her clothes and carrying her bag, when eating, drinking, consuming and tasting, when shitting and pissing, when walking, standing, sitting, falling asleep, waking up, talking, and keeping silent... (Ñāṇamoli and Bodhi, 1995:147).

This meditation is not restricted to awareness of one's own body, but includes being aware of others' bodies too. One attends to their poignant physical presence, the way others inhabit and move their bodies, the way their bodies interact with yours, the way their eyes and mouths signal emotion, pleasure, pain, fear, longing, love, hate, the way their hand squeezes yours, the way you press against each other as you embrace.

Embodied meditation does not shy away from peeling off the skin and imagining what lies inside the body either. One scans the body "up from the soles of the feet and down from the top of the head", recollecting the "head-hairs, body-hairs, nails, teeth, skin, flesh, sinews, bones, bone-marrow, kidneys, heart, liver, diaphragm, spleen, lungs, intestines, stomach contents, feces, bile, phlegm, pus, blood, sweat, fat, tears, grease, spittle, snot, oil of the joints, and urine." In Gotama's day, wanderers would meditate in charnel grounds, observing corpses as they became "bloated, livid and oozing matter" as they were torn apart and devoured by crows, jackals, and worms. "This body too", they would reflect, "is of the same nature, it will be like that, it is not exempt from that fate" (Ñāṇamoli and Bodhi, 1995: 148). To be mindful of the body involves an honesty and courage to go beyond the revulsion one may feel about its constituent parts and the terror invoked by anticipation of its death and disintegration.

The transformative power of Gotama's teaching originates in opening one's heart and mind unconditionally to the everyday sublime. One starts with what is most close and intimate: the body itself. Then one turns this attention to the hedonic tonality of one's experience, the entire spectrum of how one feels in a given situation at a given moment. These feelings, too, are initially registered in the flesh: an uneasiness in the stomach, a warmth and openness in the chest, a constriction in the throat, a stirring in the genitals. At this point the affective dimension of meditation comes into play. While mindfulness entails a degree of detachment and equanimity, this is not a cold, disinterested state of mind. To know fully the shades and nuances of one's feelings, one needs first to quieten the inner turmoil so often provoked by them in order to establish a clear, penetrating attention. Cultivating such awareness of feelings is crucial because many habitual reactive patterns are triggered as much by these subjective bodily affects as by the objects or persons we believe to be responsible for them. I might react with fear to another person's threat of violence, but that instinctive reaction is prompted by the way I feel about what has been said, which is registered somewhere in my body. Mindfulness allows us to open up a gap between his angry words and my feelings about them, which usually appear so fused together that they are hard to disentangle. In nurturing this gap, one learns how to dwell calmly and vividly in its space, which, I would argue, is the "clearly visible, immediate and inviting" space of nirvana itself (Bodhi, 2012: 919).

The Buddhist tradition presents the cultivation of mindfulness along a spectrum that starts with a fairly narrow attention to one's breath and expands into a comprehensive awareness of whatever is occurring in one's body, mind and environment. In the *Satipaṭṭhāna Sutta*, the classic presentation of mindfulness in the Pali Canon, this practice culminates in the Four Tasks themselves. It would be a mistake, however, to think that one should meditate on these tasks in the same way as one would pay attention to the breath or the body. Here, *sati* should be understood in its more literal meaning of "recollection" rather than "mindfulness." I take this to mean that the practice of mindfulness includes *recollecting* the core ideas of Gotama's teaching as a way of further refining one's awareness of experience as a whole.

"What is the power of mindfulness?" asks Gotama in another *sutta*. "Here a disciple is mindful; he is equipped with the keenest mindfulness and awareness; he recollects well and keeps in mind *what has been said and done in the past*" (Bodhi, 2012: 637, my emphasis). To be mindful of the breath, for example, means first to recollect an instruction heard in the past—whether ten minutes or ten years ago—and then to apply it by sustaining one's attention on the breath. If the attention wanders off, this means that I have forgotten what I was supposed to be doing, and thus need to remind myself again. This is not dissimilar to the kind of recollective awareness one has of being a married person, which, though largely unconscious, will trigger awareness of one's marriage vows as soon as one's thoughts stray to doing something in conflict with them. This 'recollective' aspect is obscured as soon as mindfulness is understood as simply being fully attentive in the present moment or remaining in a state of non-judgmental awareness, neither of which would seem to have much to do with remembering something said or done in the past.

To ground mindfulness in the Four Tasks means to keep these ideas in mind and apply them to illuminate whatever is taking place in one's experience at a given time and place. In this way, the Four Tasks serve as a framing device that provides meditation with its raison d'être. From this perspective, the aim of meditation is to cultivate a way of life (fourth task) rooted in consciously valorizing experiences of stopping (third task) that are brought about by the letting go of self-centred craving (second task), which, in turn, is a consequence of embracing the everyday sublime (first task). When the *Satipaṭṭhāna Sutta* describes mindfulness as the "one path to nirvana", it affirms how paying radical attention to life leads to a falling away of habitual patterns, which leads to nirvanic moments when we realize the freedom to respond to life unconditioned by our longings and fears, which opens up the possibility of living more sanely in this world. Nirvana is not reached through sustained non-conceptual concentration on a privileged religious object, but by paying close, uncompromising attention to our fluctuating, anguished bodies and minds.

The Noble Quest

The Buddha described what he awakened to as clearly visible (*sandit-thiko*), but hard to see (*dudaso*). In *The Noble Quest*, he states how this awakening was an existential shift from a frame of mind in which he "loved, delighted and reveled in his place" (Ñāṇamoli and Bodhi, 1995:260) to one in which he beheld his 'ground', which consisted of the sheer contingency of his life, on one hand, and the nirvanic suspension of self-interested craving, on the other. While both these 'grounds' are clearly visible, and thus, in a sense, self-evident, they are difficult to see because our view of them tends to be obscured by our attachments to what we identify as our place in the world. Not surprisingly, people prefer the security of something apparently solid and real than the vertiginous and bewildering play of contingency, and find it easier to react to moral dilemmas by following the prompts of their habitual self-interest, greed, and hatred than the ethical uncertainty of having to respond in ways that are not determined by them.

The 'clearly visible' nature of the dharma puzzled the wanderer 'Top-knot' Sīvaka and prompted him to ask the Buddha to explain what he meant. Gotama turns to him and says:

> Well then, Sīvaka, I will question you about this. Answer as you see fit. What do you think, Sīvaka? When there is greed within you, do you know: 'there is greed within me,' and when there is no greed within you, do you know: 'there is no greed within me'? [The same question is then repeated with 'hatred' and 'confusion' instead of 'greed']. (Bodhi, 2012: 919)

Sīvaka replies that, yes, he is able to make such a distinction. So, it is in just this way, continues Gotama, that "the Dharma is clearly visible, immediate, inviting one to come and see, applicable, to be personally known by the wise" (ibid).

In the maieutic style of a Socratic dialogue or Zen koan, Gotama draws out the answer to Sīvaka's question by having Sīvaka probe into his own first-hand experience. As Sīvaka was not a Buddhist, to see the dharma clearly cannot be an exclusive privilege of those who are committed to Buddhism. This perspective on life is available to anyone who is prepared to pay mindful, unsentimental attention to certain features of their experience. Such a perspective is "immediate" (*akaliko*): it is not the product of a gradual process of reflection and meditation over time, but is evident here and now. The dharma is also "inviting" (*ehipassiko*). This suggests that contingency and nirvana already hold an intuitive appeal as the barely audible call of your own most authentic ground. And the dharma is "applicable" (*opanayiko*): it is something to be taken up and put into practice. It is not a doctrine, or set of doctrines, to believe or disbelieve in, but something to do, which can have a direct effect on how one lives in and experience this world.

It almost sounds too easy. The dharma was accessible to Sīvaka as soon as he recognized the presence or absence of greed, hatred, and confusion within his own mind. The figure of Sīvaka stands for the perplexed everyman; he is no different from you and me. To know for oneself how these powerful drives that incline one to think and act according to their imperatives are sometimes active and sometimes not is already a glimpse of nirvana, wherein lies the source of one's freedom. In another dialogue, the Buddha tells the brahmin Jānussoṇī how a person who has let go of greed, hatred, and confusion "neither plans for his own harm, nor for the harm of others, nor for the harm of both; and he does not experience in his mind suffering and grief. In this way, brahmin, nirvana is clearly visible, immediate, inviting one to come and see, applicable, to be personally experienced by the wise" (Bodhi, 2012: 253).

As a key element in this process of awakening, the practice of mindfulness is a constant challenge to live one's life from the perspective of a groundless ground of nirvanic contingency instead of the superficially consoling convictions of one's place. Such a groundless ground is simultaneously fascinating and terrifying; it both intrigues and unsettles you. It is nothing other than the everyday sublime.

As soon as we start considering meditation from an ethical and existential perspective, we realize the inadequacy of thinking of it as primarily a cognitive process. We likewise recognize how untenable it is to think of awakening as just an enhanced kind of knowing. That mindfulness includes a cognitive dimension, however, is quite clear: for the meditator systematically focuses her/his attention on features of experience that are habitually overlooked or denied, thus cultivating a cognition of impermanence, for example, rather than persisting in an assumption of permanence. Yet in coming to know intimately the impermanent, tragic and empty aspects of life, one also opens oneself to unsuspected affective and aesthetic possibilities of experience.

In addition to paying refined attention to the spectrum of feelings and mental states that arise 'inside' (*ajjhatta*) oneself, the *Satipaṭṭhāna Sutta* states that one pay attention to feelings and mental states that occur 'outside' (*bahiddhā*) oneself as well. This is a clear indication that the cultivation of mindfulness extends beyond the boundaries of one's own skin to the feelings and mental states of other people and living organisms. I take this to mean that the development of awareness in the context of the Four Tasks entails a fundamental realignment of one's sensitivity to the feelings, needs, longings, and fears of others. Rather than requiring a supersensory capacity to 'read' other people's minds, this is a call to empathize with the condition and plight of others as revealed through an enhanced 'reading' of their bodies, which comes from the stilling and brightening of one's own awareness through meditative discipline. Making mindfulness other-centered disrupts the innate tendencies of egoism, and thus contributes to the second task of letting go of self-interested craving.

In European languages such as French, Italian, Spanish, and German, a distinction is made between a *cognitive* and *affective* knowing. In French, for example, one distinguishes between *savoir* (to know facts) and *connaître* (to know people). As mindfulness matures, it extends from knowing such facts of life as transience and suffering with greater clarity, to knowing transient and suffering people with greater empathy and sensitivity. Furthermore, as *connaître* is also used to denote how one 'knows' a piece of music, a book, a play, a landscape, a town, or a path, its kind of knowing comes to assume an aesthetic, as well as an affective, force.

Mindfulness and Modernity

The introduction of mindfulness into a secular context risks reducing it to a problem-solving technique. However effective this might prove to be in alleviating aspects of human suffering, one can lose sight of how mindful awareness concerns not just attending to specific problems in one's own life, but to life in its totality. Meditation is not only a solution to a particular set of problems, but a way of penetrating into the mystery that there is anything at all rather than nothing. When a problem is solved, it disappears, but when a mystery is penetrated, it only becomes more mysterious. In this sense, mindfulness serves as a doorway into a way of life that embraces the overwhelming totality of what it means to be a sentient human creature.

A secular approach to Buddhism could likewise unwittingly encourage the same tendency to regard meditation as a method for solving problems. By stripping away all overt elements of religious behavior and belief from the dharma, Secular Buddhism—as it is now being called—could also end up rejecting any sense of sublimity, mystery, awe, or wonder from the practice. This tendency is further reinforced when meditation is presented by its enthusiasts as a "science of the mind"; people are routinely wired up to functional magnetic resonance imaging scanners to take detailed readings of brain function while meditating, and government-sponsored studies are conducted on volunteers over long periods in order to understand the "effectiveness" of meditation. While I have no objections to any of this research as such, and acknowledge that it could provide valuable information about meditation and its effects on the human brain, the language used and imagery evoked are highly suggestive of the "technologization" of meditative practice.

Nor am I persuaded by the oft-heard complaint among traditional Buddhists that the mindfulness movement is a 'dumbing down' of the dharma. This strikes me as an elitist objection that fails to recognize how, in practice, Buddhism has been dumbing itself down ever since it began. I doubt that those who condemn the mindfulness movement on such grounds would likewise condemn the practice of millions of Buddhists that consists of repeating the name of a mythical Buddha or the title of a revered scripture. Mindfulness is becoming the *Om Mani Padme Hum* of Secular Buddhism. Yet, instead of mumbling a mantra while spinning a prayer wheel and going to the monastery once a week to offer butter lamps, today's equivalent is to sit for twenty minutes a day on a cushion observing one's breath and once a week attend a 'sitting group' in a friend's living room. In both cases, those involved may have little understanding of the subtleties of Buddhist philosophy or doctrine, but find these simple exercises deeply rewarding in helping them live balanced and meaningful lives.

In retrospect, the widespread adoption of mindfulness in diverse areas of contemporary life may come to be seen as part of the longer historical process of Buddhism's adaptation to modernity. It might mark a key moment in the acceptance of contemplative disciplines in a secular context, thus transforming the public perception of meditation from an exotic, alien, and marginal practice into an unexceptional and mainstream activity. If this turns out to be the case, then rather than complain about the 'dumbing down' of the dharma, Buddhists need to rise to the challenge of articulating a philosophically coherent and ethically integrated vision of life that is no longer tied to the religious dogmas and institutions of Asian Buddhism. In this way, perhaps, they might help encourage the dawning of a culture of awakening, which may or may not call itself 'Buddhist.'

References

Batchelor, S. (2012) 'A Secular Buddhism', *Journal of Global Buddhism*, 13, 87–107.
Bodhi, B. (2000) *The Connected Discourses of the Buddha* (Boston, MA: Wisdom Publications).
Bodhi, B. (2012) *The Numerical Discourses of the Buddha* (Somerville, MA: Wisdom Publications).
Ñāṇamoli, B. and Bodhi B. (1995) *The Middle Length Discourses of the Buddha*, Bhikkhu (Boston, MA: Wisdom Publications).
Wittgenstein, L. (1961). Tr. Pears and McGuinness *Tractatus Logico Philosophicus* (London: Routledge).

4
Mindfulness: A Philosophical Assessment

David Brazier

The Problem

The idea of mindfulness has achieved a surprisingly extensive following, but what is mindfulness? In the Buddhist texts the word is used in a range of ways. At one end of the spectrum, mindfulness can be synonymous with awareness. "Whether he inhale a long breath, let him be conscious thereof; or whether he exhale a long breath, let him be conscious thereof. Whether he inhale a short breath, or exhale a short breath, let him be conscious thereof" (Rhys Davids 1966: 328). Here mindfulness implies conscious and deliberate investigation of what one is doing, or, perhaps we should say, of what is going on in one. This is the meaning of mindfulness for the beginner. At the other end of the spectrum, for the more advanced practitioner, mindfulness refers either to deep understanding, especially of the key doctrines of Buddhism, or to recollection of wholesome objects. These latter two do, of course, to an extent, coincide as the key doctrines are themselves wholesome objects and, conversely, wholesome objects are always amenable to ever deeper understanding.

The simple meaning of mindfulness as a term in English is "to keep something in mind", and this serves quite well. One can, therefore, discern a variety of mindfulnesses according to what it is that is supposed to be kept in mind. In particular, we can distinguish those who promote (a) keeping the mind in the present moment; (b) being on one's guard and remembering not to be taken in by superficial appearances; (c) keeping in mind a deeper meaning to life than the everyday; (d) 'seeing deeply', by which is meant seeing the past origins and future destiny of what is encountered; (e) awareness of the social, economic, or political context of events, among others. Clearly, these are not all the same thing.

Is mindfulness a matter of cultivating a sharper awareness of what is immediately presented to the senses, or is it an ability to put such data in perspective? If the latter, which particular perspective? If the former, which data in particular, given that it is not possible to be consciously aware of everything that the senses are picking up? One can readily see that many different answers to these questions could be given, and among them would figure a number of different options that might sometimes have beneficial or therapeutic effect, being con-ducive to emotional stability or ability to make sound judgments, or assist performance of various tasks. There would also be options that, in certain contexts, would be dysfunctional or counter-productive. So a further question arises regarding where and when particular forms of mindfulness might be appropriate or useful.

As we try to penetrate into the subject conceptually, it is apparent that there is no single universal definition of mindfulness. When I was studying mind and cognition with Tibetan teachers, I was taught that the mind is clear and cognizing. This meant that a mind always has an object. To say the same thing differently, we are always mindful of some-thing. If we are always inherently mindful of something, advocacy of mindfulness as such is redundant. What becomes salient, as seen above, is the question: Mindfulness of what? There is a danger that the term mindfulness provides an umbrella under which just about anything can be advocated.

Consciousness and Deliberation

An even more fundamental critique is also available. There seems to be implicit in the notion of mindfulness the idea that we are talking about conscious awareness. To keep something in mind implies deliberation. Is advocacy of mindfulness really an updated advocacy of consciousness? If so, then we have to ask whether extending consciousness is necessarily always a good thing.

Clearly, human beings are not conscious all the time. Some of the time we are asleep. Sleep performs a vitally important function. During sleep we may dream. Dreaming is a mode of consciousness, but not one that is necessarily remembered. Is one being mindful while dreaming? If we say not, we must, nonetheless, allow that dreaming performs a useful function. Approximately one third of the time of a human life is taken up by sleep. This non-mindful time is vital to health.

What about the other two thirds? How about day-dreaming? From time to time, fantasies invade the mind. Is this wasted time? Should we train ourselves to eliminate this phenomenon? At school we are taught to concentrate on our lessons and not sit dreaming of playing football instead. Learning to concentrate is certainly useful and has its place. However, day-dreaming also has its uses and delights. Should it be eliminated? Surely not. Such times provide rest and recuperation from stress. They can also prove to be creative. These are times when intuitions have access to the mind. Along with actual sleep, they are times when deeper layers of the mind are able to process data. We are all aware of the phenomenon of having a problem that we cannot solve to which an answer later occurs as from nowhere. There are aspects of the mind that function better when released from conscious control.

Related to this notion of the value of the free-wheeling mind is the role of play. Play has a greater element of consciousness in it than day-dreaming, but it is still a mode in which the mind is largely under the sway of fantasy. Play should not just be for children. It is surely an essential element in the achievement of a balanced life. Adults do not play enough. Perhaps this is why they tend to become habituated to consciousness-reducing or tranquilizing drugs and recreational substances. The craving to be released from full consciousness is strong.

What I am saying is that the natural and healthily functioning human being is in a state of at least reduced consciousness for at least two thirds of the time, and that this time is not to be considered wasted. We certainly cannot, therefore, advocate twenty-four-hour-a-day mindfulness as a desirable practice.

Awareness and Wariness

So is mindfulness about sharpening awareness at the times when conscious awareness is appropriate? What are those times? And when we say sharpening, what do we mean?

Perhaps we have to begin by asking what conscious awareness is for. Awareness is connected with wariness. Wariness has survival value. It is useful for hunting and for avoiding becoming prey. In a dangerous world, intelligence and awareness work together to enable one to foresee opportunities, devise strategies, avoid pitfalls, seize what one needs, and escape.

It is surely on the back of these abilities that we have developed a number of traits that we now consider to be virtues. The ability to empathize, for instance, rests on our ability to understand another creature and foresee its actions. Out of raw instincts evolved for killing and avoiding being killed we have developed skills in caring. Less evolved animals simply laid their eggs and went away. Mammals and birds care for their young. Social animals may even care for those to whom they are not closely related.

The human project seems to be to go beyond our nature and develop traits that raise us to a higher and more enlightened level of collective life. We are doing this using the raw materials of instinct originally developed for less elevated purposes.

We need to bear in mind, however, that simply being aware of something carries no moral implication. It makes perfectly good sense to say, 'He mindfully pulled the trigger, and watched the blood splatter from the child's head as its body slumped to the ground.' It is possible to fall into the mistake of thinking that an act carries no karmic consequence if carried out in the correct state of mind. This, however, can be a very dangerous doctrine that would not need mention if it had not, from time to time in history, facilitated terrible atrocities.

Stress Reduction

The popularity of mindfulness is linked to its supposed power to reduce stress. Undoubtedly, there are ways to reduce stress, and some of these could fall under the heading of mindfulness. Should mindfulness, then, be defined as the things that reduce stress?

The principal way to reduce stress is to relax. Certain relaxation techniques can be learnt. Most of these involve directing attention to particular parts of the body. If I direct my attention to my toes, especially if I imagine that I am just about to curl them or move them in some other way, my body will direct a slightly larger quantity of blood to the area in preparation for the action. This enhanced blood supply will have a cleansing effect, removing some toxins from the muscles. If I then continue the exercise and do a complete body scan, muscle group by muscle group, I may succeed in reducing the amount of toxins from muscles in many parts of my body. This may successfully reverse the previous toxin inducing effect of stress.

Again, if I simply keep my attention on my feet and not allow it to move to other parts, this may temporarily deprive the upper part of my body of its full blood supply and may induce sleep, which will also have a stress reducing effect. These types of techniques used to be called relaxation exercises, but nowadays may be classified under mindfulness. Clearly, they can be useful in appropriate circumstances. I have certainly found them helpful while sitting in the dentist's waiting room. Whether this has much, if anything, to do with mindfulness as described in the Buddhist sutras, however, is an open question.

Rationalism

In the eighteenth and nineteenth centuries we collectively experienced something called the Enlightenment. This centered upon an attempt to raise rationalism to a high status. It yielded science and industry, enabled the human population to multiply tenfold, some diseases to be banished, home comforts to be developed, and all the benefits of technology to become ours.

This achievement certainly involved an extension of consciousness, though not generally of the present moment awareness type. It was the development of logic, empiricism, planning, and control.

We have now moved into a post-enlightenment phase. Some call this post-modernism. Technology is still advancing, especially in the fields of electronics and biology. Life remains fundamentally a mystery. Nobody has managed to manufacture it from inanimate chemicals in a test tube nor have we yet discovered it anywhere else in the cosmos. The huge population of humans that now inhabits Earth has begun to feel insecure, seeing its own burgeoning destroying the environment upon which it depends and, as yet, having nowhere else to go. To survive, it appears that the species is going to have to evolve a level of collective self-restraint not previously accomplished. Does mindfulness have a part to play in this? Are we seeing a new need for wariness?

Here and Now

Let's go back to the definition. I have said that, in one sense, we are always mindful anyway inasmuch as the mind is always full of something, even if it is in sleep or fantasy. To define mindfulness we need to say what it is not. Generally, it will be said that the two thirds of life when we are asleep or ruminating are not times of mindfulness in the narrower sense. How narrow should we go?

One current common definition of mindfulness talks about dwelling in the present moment. It is said, rhetorically, that only the present moment exists, the past having passed away and the future not yet arrived. This may sound profound, but is surely only tautology. There is really no reason to think any particular moment more or less real than any other. Further, the here and now, for me, is only such because it is where I am at this moment. In other words, it is defined by my presence. If all that is real in this universe is defined as such by my presence then have I not fallen into the most complete form of solipsism?

When I was young, to say that somebody lived in the here and now meant that they were irresponsible—a proper concern for the future and an ability to reflect upon the past being essential ingredients of maturity. Is mindfulness a form of regression to a childlike innocence? Surely the mind is equipped to scan the past, present, and future in a seamlessly integrated way, and this is hardly something that can be taken apart. If I try to practice here and now awareness, I am still doing something at the same time. Let us say that I am setting the table for lunch, putting out cutlery and utensils. If I have done my mindfulness training, then I will be now more than formerly aware of the texture of the vessels, the shininess of the cutlery, the disposition of the various objects. This may increase my aesthetic appreciation of the scene and yield a certain satisfaction. All the time, however, my mind is simultaneously making small decisions, drawing on past experience and directing muscular action that is future oriented. Really, there is no such thing as the present moment. Time is a flow and mind is in that flow.

Distraction and Unconscious Process

Consciousness is specific. Mindfulness of one thing means withdrawing attention from something else. This is why being in the here and now was regarded as irresponsible by my grandparents. If one were only thinking about the present, then one was not remembering one's various duties. To give some trite examples, if I really live in the here and now, I will not read the newspapers and I will certainly not concern myself with the plight of those suffering in far off places, nor shall I make provision for tomorrow. Those who live in the here and now should not go shopping.

This, of course, is not what contemporary advocates of mindfulness have in mind, but is it actually possible to say what mindfulness is not? If only the present moment is real, then our anticipation of the future and concern with the past must be admitted to take place in the present moment and so be as real as anything else. But if everything is included in the present moment, then it becomes redundant to advocate being there as we have no choice anyway. The whole subject runs the danger of becoming trivially true and empty of real content.

At any moment the mind is fixed on an object, though generally only momentarily. Mostly, the senses are engaged in scanning, picking up large quantities of fragmentary data out of which the brain then constructs coherent pictures. Some of these pictures are visual, some are patterns of sound, some relate to other sense modes. They give an illusion of here and now-ness, but what we see as here and now is actually a construction from a linear sequence of impressions collected over time. This is how we make sense of our world. This is more obviously apparent with sound than sight. Sounds, clearly, are not just momentary. They make sense as a sequence.

Is mindfulness, then, really not 'being in the here and now,' but rather entering the flow? If it is, does it really depend on sharp consciousness?

If I am playing tennis, mindfulness means to keep my eye on the ball. I see the ball coming, see it connect with my racquet; see it speed into the other court. This is not all that I am doing, of course. At the same time as I am watching the ball, my feet have moved to new positions; my hand has tightened its grip on the handle; my shoulders, arms, hips, and torso have demonstrated the complicated versatility needed to bring the head of the racquet into contact with the ball at exactly the right moment, angle, and velocity. In other words, the bulk of the maneuvre has been done outside of my direct awareness. Indeed, if my awareness had gone to what my feet were doing I would have missed the ball.

The possibility arises, therefore, that mindfulness plays a double role. On the one hand, keeping my eye on the ball does gather information. On the other hand, keeping my attention there also functions as a distraction technique necessary to keep the conscious mind out of the way while the unconscious dimensions of the mind do their work. When we consider this example, it is clear that the unconscious element is considerably larger and more complex than the conscious one.

This, therefore, gives us a rather different picture of how the human organism functions. The greater part is unconscious or autonomic. These hidden elements are partly instinctive and partly trainable, but when they are functioning they do so without much conscious control. At most, consciousness is like a sheep dog rounding up a large flock of sheep. The unconscious—the sheep—is what matters and the sheepdog cannot be on duty all the time. Further, it is sometimes necessary to keep the sheepdog out of the way so that the sheep can get on with doing all the things that they know how to do perfectly well without interference.

Where does this leave us with mindfulness? First, it seems that the term is open to a number of meanings and so it will be important when examining the claims of particular methodologies or pieces of research to first clarify what is actually being referred to. Second, it may well be that the mechanism by which much mindfulness achieves the effects it does has a good deal to do with its function as a distraction that enables stressful material to be avoided or unconscious processes to continue unhindered.

Mindfulness in Buddhism 1: In the *Satipaṭṭhāna Sutta*

So what does mindfulness mean in Buddhism? Let us take Buddhism to be a path of liberation through finding out the truth. In the introduction I wrote that there were preliminary forms of mindfulness—"Whether he inhale a long breath, let him be conscious thereof; or whether he exhale a long breath, let him be conscious thereof. Whether he inhale a short breath, or exhale a short breath, let him be conscious thereof" (Rhys Davids 1966:328)—and more advanced forms in which one had in mind the truths of the dharma. These are references to the *Satipaṭṭhāna Sutta*. In the beginning of the *Sutta* we find exercises of immediate awareness, first of bodily movement, then of feelings, then of emotions. By the end of the *Sutta* it is talking about awareness of the Four Truths for Noble Ones and other important Buddhist doctrines. How does this fit together?

I think the key is that this is about investigation. The truths of the dharma are not intellectual propositions so much as formulations of the facts of life and existence. They are to know that things are impermanent, mind is conditioned, we are mortal, bad things happen, a noble life is possible nonetheless, and so on, but not just to know these things as information or facts, but to know them through experience.

Mindfulness, in this context means *experiential learning*. Studying the breath, one learns directly that there is a limit to one's control over it, that it ultimately regulates itself, that it fluctuates in a manner conditioned by other things happening in one's body and mind, and so on. Studying the emotions one sees that they come and go, that we can do a certain amount to regulate them, but also that they seem to have a life of their own. We see that they do not conform to our idealistic notions of how we think we should be. Mindfulness, in this context, means facing reality and seeing the truth about ourselves for ourselves.

Although there were health benefits, including some stress reduction, these are clearly not the prime aim of the *Sutta*. Buddha was not advocating a health cure. Any benefit of that kind was incidental. Rather, he wanted us to know the truth about ourselves. Mindfulness, in this *Sutta*, is a program of looking in order to find out.

Mindfulness in Buddhism 2: In the Seven Enlightenment Factors

Mindfulness is one of the seven factors of awakening. We can see these seven as the foundation for all therapy. They prescribe that therapy should be conducted in a place of peace, in a state of rapture, with a focus upon a courageous investigation of truth which should be comprehended with one's whole being, which is to say, mindfully.

The Indian word *smṛti* (*sati* in Pali) comes from the root meaning *to remember*. Buddhism is a matter of waking up and this implies that what we realize is something that has been there all along. Smṛti is an *anamnesis*—a remembering. We have known all this before. The experience of awakening to the dharma is more a recognition than a new cognition. Like waking up in the morning, one gradually comes to consciousness and recognizes one's surroundings, remembers who one is and what one must do. Maybe, like Buddha himself, one is initially reluctant, but then one's energy rises and one goes forth into the day. Similarly, spiritual awakening sends one forth into the world, for the good of the many, for the benefit of gods and humans. We have been free all along, but we were not willing to see that freedom. Liberation is awakening to our freedom and therapy is a path toward such awakening, a path in which one accompanies another.

If Buddhism is an awakening through direct experience to our essential freedom, it is not just a matter of living in the here and now; it encompasses the whole of life. In the sutras we see the Buddha capable of reminiscing and planning, and of making provision for people not present. He saw the value of not worrying about what might well not happen, but to say that the key to understanding his approach is to live in the here and now is going too far. In particular, the Buddha liked to remember his own experience of awakening. Calling it to mind no doubt gave him strength. This fits well with our understanding of mindfulness as experiential learning, learning of things that will be of great value and see one through the difficulties of life.

Experiential Learning, not a Treatment

The effect of experiential learning is that one knows things by experience and not simply as conceptual knowledge. Buddha pointed out various truths, but he did not want people just to learn what he said; he wanted them to have the experiences that would make such knowledge real for them. When it was real they would have it. They would not necessarily be conscious of it all the time, but it would be so much a part of them that they would act upon it whenever appropriate.

From a Buddhist point of view, then, mindfulness is not really a treatment. The modern usage has taken mindfulness to be a treatment, as if it were a kind of medical application. Whereas for Buddha mindfulness is a means of finding out something important. To ask and research 'the effects of mindfulness' is not wholly unlike researching the effects of thinking or looking or searching. That would surely be a case of what the Buddha called picking up the snake at the wrong end.

Reducing something like mindfulness to a technique or a treatment is a stage in the decline of the dharma. As Buddha advocates it, mindfulness is about finding out and becoming liberated. When we are liberated, life is more spontaneous and unpredictable. We are in the flow. When mindfulness becomes a treatment or a technique, it is done with a predetermined aim in view and that is not what liberation means.

What are we Looking for?

Mindfulness is part of the Buddha's advocacy that one should really find out what is true for oneself by one's own experience. He is saying look carefully! He taught that finding the truth for oneself is what liberates people. If one knows for oneself, then one can make one's own decisions in life. He was not interested in making people into slavish followers. He was interested in helping them to equip themselves to live their lives in as real a manner as possible because they had investigated the real world for themselves.

The real world is not the ideal world. It is not a single desirable state that can be attained by the application of a procedure. In our investigation we may discover what we are. What we are will not accord with our various ideals. It will include the presence in us of many different emotions, some more laudable than others. It will include our attachment to unfinished business from our past, and all manner of pride, dejection, greed, aversion, sloth, worry, and fragility. We are human, mortal, and vulnerable.

Knowing these things we shall want to do something about some of them. We will feel shame and want to change some things. Liberation is, however, not primarily about becoming more moral as such. It is about having the choice and the ability to do so because one knows the truth. This truth may include knowledge that there are some things one can do nothing about and some things one can change. To be liberated is to know and to choose where choice is possible and to deeply accept where change is not possible.

The Future

Where, then, does this leave us with the current vogue for mindfulness methods? Clearly, mindfulness as a treatment method is different from mindfulness as a means of investigation. Nonetheless, it is currently popular and does include some techniques that do help people in some specific situations. Mindfulness has become an ensign under which many ships can sail, some of which carry good cargo. As currently applied, the concept lacks coherence and is rather wide of its meaning in its original Buddhist context, but that does not mean that all is lost. Mindfulness is, in a sense, as I once heard Stephen Batchelor remark, a kind of Trojan horse, smuggling a variety of Buddhist ways of thinking into popular culture. Whether Buddhism itself is becoming distorted in the process is something that we shall not see clearly until much later.

The range of supposedly 'mindfulness-based' offerings is steadily increasing. In the process, the term is losing whatever specificity of definition it may once have had. This, however, is a normal phase in any such dissemination. I have some familiarity with the work of Carl Rogers, whom I knew many years ago. Once the ideas of Carl Rogers were considered revolutionary and the definitions of his works were tight. However, as the idea of being client- or person-centered became widespread, it soon came to mean whatever people wanted it to mean and was watered down to a point close to meaninglessness. The same will happen with mindfulness. Just as everything involving persons can, at a stretch, be called person-centered, so everything involving minds can be termed mindful. Of course, something is lost in the process, but then those who do things rigorously are always few.

Nonetheless, along the way, some good things will have happened. Some people will have been helped, some people will have learnt some things about Buddhism, some therapists will have thought about their work in new ways. No doubt, usage will go on evolving. The original meaning will not go away. The Buddhist texts will still be there to refer to, and from time to time somebody may recover the original meaning and benefit from it. Again, the spiritual path unfolds in paradoxical ways. This is because, by definition, we are not enlightened before we start. We naturally approach the matter in a deluded way. Our initial reasons for practicing are to do with ambition, search for comfort, desire for freedom from particular sufferings or fears, or simple envy of others who seem to have something we have not got. None of these kinds of motives are pure nor are they likely to bring good results directly. Nonetheless, the fact that we practise at all means that we keep ourselves broadly within a domain where we may stumble upon the truth by accident.

Actually, this is commonly how the truth reveals itself to us. Paradoxically, it comes at just those times when we were not fully conscious, not on guard, not wary. It is worth making an effort at mindfulness, but it will be just at the point where one's mindfulness fails that something of interest may really pop up.

Reference

Rhys Davids, T. W. (1966) *Dialogues of the Buddha, Part 2* (London: Luzac).

5
Mindfulness and the Good Life

Manu Bazzano

Dedicated to Mark Payge (1950–2013)

Introducing Embodied Dharma Practice

There are forty things worth remembering, the Buddha says in his *Discourse on the Foundation of Mindfulness* (Thera, 1973). Top of the list are the certainty of death and the uncertainty of the time of its occurrence. What is worth remembering is that this mysterious, dazzling, and tumultuous life—this life we fear and cherish—blooms right into the arms of death. Similarly, the great Tibetan poet and scholar Gendun Chöpel (2009) reminds us that the riches of the world are mist on a mountain pass. Our closest friends are like guests on market day.

Dharma practitioners of all persuasions call this state of affairs 'impermanence.' Mindfulness is first and foremost *mindfulness of impermanence*. It is tempting to liken this awareness to a melancholy insight, a sentiment, a *mood* even—but that would be inaccurate. Instead, we are asked to acquire a simple yet profound sensibility, and to allow this sensibility to affect us to the core. What we then may come to perceive in the heart of life is the delicate and pitiless work of death. We notice flux and transformation; we feel the very current of 'living-and-dying' (*shōji*—one word in the Zen tradition, not two, denoting two sides of the same coin).

This unflinching gaze on the essentially tragic nature of human existence singles out dharma teachings from the glistening platitudes of the *new age*, from the otherworldly ambience of various 'transpersonal' approaches to psychology and spirituality, and from the remedial array of positivist techniques now in vogue. Often confused with one or all of the above, what I call *embodied dharma practice* steers an altogether different course: it is a path away from consolation and towards a deeper appreciation of life.

Walking on Hell, Gazing at Flowers

If the teachings of the Buddha were only a *memento mori*, solely indicating our finitude, there would be, perhaps, no substantial difference between embodied dharma practice and the Judaeo–Christian tradition (at least not in the way in which the latter has been assimilated in mainstream Western culture). There would be no need, as Jung (1962) rather melodramatically complained, to be misled by the devil by going in search of Eastern occultism and yoga practices. We would be much better off rediscovering our Western tradition without ever bothering to venture east.

However, the teachings of the Buddha cannot be confused with 'Eastern occultism' (or with Western 'spirituality') because they invite us to step beyond the sad realization of life's transience. This invitation is neatly summed up by the eighteenth-century haiku poet Issa when he tells us to never forget—for we walk on hell, gazing at flowers (Bazzano, 2002).

Not forgetting that life is suffering, and 'hell' all too real, goes over the familiar pious ground. But gazing at flowers comes as a surprise: it throws open the gates of 'heaven'—it does not lead us to all things pristine and everlasting, into a portentous afterlife with special effects, but invites us, instead, to a sharper perception of phenomena. It invites us to the *thusness* of things, to life as it is—as it unfolds. As it *becomes*.

Ordained to Praise

I went out early this morning. It was sunny at last after many days of rain. The florist at the corner was sweeping the ground outside his kiosk. The waitress from the café across the street stepped out to greet him loudly and cheerfully. He responded heartily and then resumed sweeping. I felt a surge of joy, unexpectedly moved by this average, yet incomparable, morning. Then joy turned to sadness. I thought of my friend Mark, who died only two weeks ago, whose funeral I attended last week, and who did not wake up to this new morning.

In the midst of life, rolling on towards death, there *are* flowers; there *is* beauty. Wayward and tentative our steps may be—our youth fleeting, our life full of mirages. Still, this evanescent world calls for our praise.

Maybe we are here to speak, to give a name to things and praise them. Like the poet, the dharma apprentice is *ordained to praise* this ephemeral world. She is exhorted to go past the all-too-familiar resentment that is our common rejoinder to the uncertainty of life. Some have argued that therapy and religion are born out of this basic resentment. If so, one is then obliged to ask: What would a religious practice or a therapeutic orientation be like that is *not* founded on resentment? Issa's "gazing at flowers" provides us with more than a hint: exposed to the ever-present reality of death in the midst of life, he asks us to sing the praises of this transient and often deeply unjust world.

'Praise' does not necessarily mean positive thinking or positive psychology—least of all contractual or guilt-ridden obligation to grate-fulness. It denotes, instead, contemplation and appreciation of the mystery of things, and the articulation of one's own unique response to that realization.

Dharma as Affirmative Art

I believe the above stance to be at variance with religions' customary displeasure with the world, a world depicted as *samsāra* in ortho-dox Buddhism and *valley of tears* in Christianity. One does find in Christianity, alongside strictly devout leanings, a lyrical and passionate acceptance of the humble and sublime pleasures of earthly living. The ardent Yea-saying of John Donne's poetry and the exaltation of earthly love in Dante (to name only two illustrious examples) are more or less easily found alongside, for instance, George Herbert's more pious rap-tures. Could it be that, still in its infancy, Western Buddhism has yet to reach the ripeness required for a spirited, life-affirming stance?

The dharma practitioner gazes at the flowers. She does not berate the world for its transience and imperfection. At the same time, she does not forget that we all walk on hell: this very ground we leisurely stroll on is the roof of the underworld, a chthonic soil peopled by innumerable dead. 'Walking mindfully' then cannot but mean walking on the frayed bones and the scattered ashes of those who came before us. It is only a matter of time until we will join them. We need to travel—or so it seems—through the horror and the sadness of this realization in order to find the inspiration for a meaningful existence.

Cultivation of mindfulness then implies a dynamic recollection of a "naked truth, terrifying to behold" (Chöpel, 2009: 47). This can work as an antidote to my own penchant for self-gratification and self-pity. These are often the trademarks of the unexamined life as a spectator in search of diversions—someone who, like me, is very keen to learn by rote the vocabulary of psychology and mindfulness.

Never forget, Issa says: countless Buddhas across the ages invite us to remember what is worth remembering. If dharma practice were an art (a craft), it could not be *narcotic* art, a Wagnerian call to deep slumber in the service of the nirvana principle (Freud, 1990) or, indeed, of the death instinct, that is, of the wish to numb our experience in order to expunge pain (obliterating our humanity in the process). It would have to be *affirmative* art (Bazzano, 2006), part of a broad *culture of awakening* (Batchelor, 1997), encouraging us to take that primary vital step of conscious resolve—a step which may turn our passivity with regards to an inescapable *fate* into active acceptance of our pliable *destiny* (Bollas, 1987).

Sex, Drugs, and the Human Soul

My client, Jim, is a keen meditator and a yoga practitioner who regularly attends intensive retreats. He came to therapy because he wanted to get his life "sorted out", as he said on our very first meeting. His successful career as a freelance designer allowed him the freedom to be creative, and gained him the respect of his clients and colleagues. He is in his mid-thirties, and married to an old friend from his university days.

His reason for coming to therapy was that he had felt his commitment to married life dwindle. He missed his former life of parties and brief romances, and a couple of times since his marriage, two and a half years ago, he had what he called "a fling." These episodes were accompanied by what he described as his 'old habits': drinking coffee and alcohol, and occasionally smoking marijuana. Although the amount he drank and smoked was small, he felt this was a problem because it ushered in what he called the "wild guy." He was also concerned that the "wild guy" was fighting a battle with the "good guy" in him. The latter would come to the fore during periods of meditation and yoga. He found it hard to meditate and do yoga regularly, but tended to go through intensive bouts, which he described as "cleansing." At these times, his body felt stronger, his mind clearer, and he would then renew his objective to be faithful to his wife, especially in view of the fact that they were planning to have children, given that, as his wife had said to him, "the clock was ticking." The desire to have children was more hers than his, though he felt he went along with it in the hope that becoming a father would help him acquire greater stability.

My own familiarity with meditation had been a deciding factor in him seeking me out. He expressed the hope that therapy would help tighten his "control over unruly behaviour", which meditation and yoga had intermittently initiated. He also anticipated that I could give him advice in terms of meditation techniques. I wanted to honour his aspirations, yet felt ambivalent, and told him so. As a therapist, I see my task as separate from that of a meditation facilitator. If someone comes to me for therapy, I respond as a therapist and refrain from being caught up in a dual role. The very notion of a 'Buddhist therapist' or even a 'mindfulness therapist' strikes me as odd. My aspiration is to be present and receptive enough to the therapeutic encounter to allow a meditative quality to be there unaided (and even undetected) for the benefit of the client. Were I to do anything more, it would strike me as prescriptive and even patronizing, as a dramatic shift from the delicate responsibility as therapist to the role of 'secular priest' and 'spiritual advisor.'

For these reasons, I did not feel compelled to interfere with Jim's meditation practice (although we did compare notes on a couple of occasions). Instead, I focused on exploring his dilemma with him. I also wanted somehow to honour, in spite of my perplexity in the matter, his aspiration to live a "good life", as he put it, and to become more of a "good guy."

The mutual affection with his wife had taken on brother–sister characteristics. He felt that his relationship with her lacked the intensity and freedom he had experienced during the last of his flings—in his own words "a very passionate, meaningful event... [which] opened me up to a parallel world... it made me feel truly alive." At the same time, he had somehow compartmentalized the experience and was not entirely comfortable exploring its fuller meaning for fear that it would "spill over" into his everyday existence and disrupt it. I discussed with my supervisor whether Jim's behavior could be seen as compulsive and its possible roots traceable in earlier narcissistic damage. Was he consciously or unconsciously choosing to anesthetize the resulting pain? Jim and I tried to explore in more detail the two facets of his life. If anything, his "wild guy" persona seemed to be endowed with a little more "soul", human vulnerability, and genuineness than the "good guy" could ever muster. The latter seemed to be strangely contrived and partly governed by a strong need for security and emotional stability. We traced this back to his parents' separation during early adolescence, a time of upheaval and uncertainty.

It emerged that both the "wild guy" and the "good guy" were dominant players in Jim's life, yet strangely failing to put him in touch with himself. The challenge was for me to hold up both aspects without implying, suggesting, or moving ahead of his own process. The positive outcome was that, to a certain extent, he managed to do the same—holding both aspects—rather than trying to eradicate one and bolster the other. He also began to see meditation as *being with* the dilemma rather than using it as a prescriptive tool in the service of a pre-existing agenda.

I chose this brief outline of my work with Jim because it is exemplary of clients who practice meditation as a way of exerting control over their emotions and affects in the pursuit of the 'good life.' The depth and breadth of questions raised is beyond the scope of this chapter, but I will outline some of the implications of this search for the good life in relation to mindfulness and meditation.

Mindfulness and 'the Good Life'

There are two ways of understanding *eudaimonia*, the good life, in the Western tradition. One, going back to Aristotle, interprets it as 'the virtuous life', clearly demarcating virtue from vice, a good deed from a bad one. A good life or a happy life (eudaimonia is often translated as 'happiness') is a virtuous life. An aberrant yet not entirely incongruous development of this perspective is the contemporary belief in 'bio-morality' (Zupancic, 2012; Bazzano, 2013a). What is bio-morality? Let me answer with the following example.

When still a trainee psychotherapist, I worked for a year as a volunteer in the renal unit of a major London hospital and also did a brief stint in palliative care. I remember it to this day as one of the most challenging jobs I've ever done. The greatest difficulty was not dealing with my general sense of inadequacy in the face of great distress, but the patients' deeply-held belief that their plight was due to having done something wrong. I can still hear my placement supervisor's mantra: "Bad things can happen to good people."

It is likewise common, in my experience, for people diagnosed with cancer to react with guilt and shame, and for their acquaintances and loved ones to link illness to various degree of wrongdoing—if not bad karma, at least bad diet. Thus, the 'virtuous life' is held up to a dutiful ideal—with deleterious results. Bio-morality means attributing physical illness and mental distress to moral shortcomings.

The other way to understand eudaimonia is to remember the *daimon* in eudaimonia—to listen to one's daimon (often confused with 'demon', in itself an intriguing Christian mis-translation). The presence of the daimon in psychic life goes back to the pre-Socratics and Greek tragedians, and it is famously mentioned by Socrates, whose wisdom is guided by the 'inner' voice of his own daimon. From the notion of the daimon, Rollo May, echoed more recently by some contemporary practitioners (Spinelli (2007) and Bazzano (2011), among others), has developed the hypothesis of the *daimonic*, which he describes as "any natural function which has the power to take over the whole person" (1969: 123). Incidentally, May's description of the daimonic as an "*archetypal* function of human experience—an *existential* reality" (ibid, my emphasis) cuts through the old Platonic (and Jungian) division between archetypes and existence. For May, being *possessed* by daimonic energies leads one to psychosis; *chastising* them, however, leads one to the anti-daimonic, which, for him, is another word for *apathy*, or absence of pathos. Could a reductive use of mindfulness do just that?

I have studied Eastern thought and practiced meditation for the last thirty-three years, all the while cherishing the belief that the Buddha's teachings do not denigrate, but *affirm*, life. I have acquired a habit along the way of applying a 'life-denigrating detector' to any philosophy, psychology, and religious practice I happen to stumble upon. The inspiration is Nietzsche, who was, in turn, inspired by Heraclitus. They both belong to an unbroken tradition—which I call, borrowing from Madison (1981), 'the counter-tradition'—which submits any system of thought or philosophical practice to a few salient questions: Does it affirm life in all its imperfection, complexity, and contradiction? Or does it look down on it, averting its gaze and directing it towards a metaphysical ideal? Does it affirm *becoming*, or does it privilege *being*? Does it affirm experience, inviting us to learn from its unfolding? Or does it postulate, instead, the existence of doctrines to which experience is subjugated? Does it *embrace* the humble joys and sorrows of ordinary, embodied human beings? Or does it disdain them as imperfect, sinful, and (a favorite word in mindfulness literature) 'unwholesome'?

The question of life-affirmation versus life denigration is central to mindfulness, a practice that (openly or covertly) amply draws on Buddhism. Is mindfulness life-affirming or life-denying? In contemporary Buddhist discourse, the question does come into view, but is disguised somewhat as a more apparent conflict between religious and secular Buddhism.

Mundane Buddhism

Secular Buddhism is not *worldly* enough. It still erects a fence between 'spiritual' practice and the world. The very origin of the term 'secular' (from *saeculum*: century) is Christian Latin, pertaining to time *in relation to* eternity, belonging to the world *in relation to* the church and religious orders, as in the term 'secular clergy.'

The term *mundane* goes one step further, meaning earthly, worldly, with no relation to the religious life, and in some languages the word is used to describe 'disreputable' professions, such as prostitution (*mondana* describes a sex worker in Italian), or 'trivial' pursuits, such as fashion and 'society life' (*vita mondana* in Italian).

There is also another important association to the word 'mundane', one that is linked to Merleau-Ponty's (1964) phenomenology (Moreira, 2012), which emphasizes the concrete, *situated* experiences of human beings in history. For Merleau-Ponty, a *mundane perspective* of human experience is intrinsically *ambiguous*, originating at the intersection of the human being and the world, taking into account the cultural, historical, and biological aspects of lived life, which together constitute "the multiple outlines of an ambiguous human development, constantly in movement" (Moreira, 2012: 56).

A secular approach to religious practice still preserves the whiff of the cloister. It frees the practitioner from transcendence, but still keeps her tied to Judaeo-Christian morality. A secular clergy will fashion itself (more or less explicitly) as morally superior to the flock. Whereas a religious Buddhist teacher will underline a vague spiritual dimension, implying, perhaps, his greater intimacy with the deities or more direct experience of enlightenment, the secular Buddhist teacher might emphasize freedom from ruminations, passions, and troublesome emotions. Both essentially chastise the contradictions and imperfections of the human condition.

I believe there are more avenues of exploration within a secular frame. My assertion has to do more with temperament and personal taste than with a belief that secularism holds a greater claim to truth. At the same time, when one scratches the surface of Protestantism (the most comprehensive and successful attempt at secularization within a major religion), one finds, perhaps, an even greater denigration of human imperfection in the name of an even sterner and prescriptive morality.

Until now, Buddhism in the West has been predominantly assimilated and interpreted within (North-American and North-European) Protestant sensibilities. There are versions of the dharma being assimilated via a southern, Catholic mentality. I am only familiar, via my short forays into Tibetan Buddhism in my early twenties, with a distinctly Catholic assimilation of a rather baroque range of deities and intricate doctrinal beliefs (karma, reincarnation, etc.). I am inclined to think, along with

James Hillman (1992), that there might be more to the 'north–south' divide than doctrinal and theological differences. Southern sensibility is polytheistic, which, in psychological terms, may translate into an appreciation of the plural nature of psyche. The south of Europe was Greek long before being Catholic. And there is more to the ancient Greeks than Plato, Socrates, and Aristotle. Long before Greek philosophy 'proper' and the establishment of its avowed unified aim, that is, *ataraxia* or imperturbability, we find the great poets/philosophers and the great tragedians inspired by Dionysus, a god symbolizing the ungraspable, the boundlessness of water, the flux of life, inexhaustible and fragmented. Finally, as strangely as it may sound to some, Dionysus is a god of *wisdom*. Euripides speaks of the wisdom of Dionysus from which philosophy itself stems. According to this interpretation, philosophy is born out of 'madness', excess, and chaos—from the full range of human life rather than from a rational and tranquil recollection of its vicissitudes.

An Appreciation of Life

I still believe that an active acceptance of the human condition runs through the Buddhist tradition. Taizan Maezumi (2001) often described the essence of Zen practice as appreciating one's life, in turn a shrewd rendering of Dōgen Zenji's 'practice/realization' being one and the same. In other words, we do not practice in order to attain realization. We practice for no reason, with no particular goal in mind. Borrowing the term from the great Latin poet Virgil (2013), who used it in relation to the craft of poetry, I call meditation an *inglorious* activity (Bazzano, 2013b).

What often happens through sustained and sincere practice, uncluttered by religious Buddhist baggage and/or secular remedial agendas, is a profound appreciation of life's givens, and the realization that life's *givens* are life's *gifts* (Bazzano, 2013c).

Appreciation is not passive acceptance of the status quo. It is not complacency. There is always room for improvement, for gaining greater freedom from hindrances, compulsions, and obfuscations—for understanding that these are often self-created. It is more helpful, however, if this is done from a stance of self-compassion rather than self-punishment. To reduce dharma practice to self-improvement is to shrink its scope to one of its possible 'side effects.' Appreciating one's life means starting from a compassionate, ironic, and active acceptance of self and others. This is not 'Buddhist resignation' but acknowledgement of the contradictions inherent in being human. The opposite stance is one of disdain, of looking down at our all too human existence in the name of transcendental and religious ideals, *or* in the name of equally lofty secular ideals. In this regard, both religious and secular Buddhism agree, even though they speak a different language.

Religious Buddhism will often juxtapose a samsaric world of greed, ignorance, and hatred to a nirvanic pure land, a static realm or an equally static 'enlightened' mental plateau.

Secular Buddhism will repeat the 'English mistake' attributed by Nietzsche to George Eliot: doing away with religious paraphernalia yet obligingly preserve its life-denying moral apparatus. It might well be that the way out of this impasse is for Buddhist practitioners to learn the lessons of contemporary ethics, which are alert to the need for a non-metaphysical, situational, and essentially radical response to otherness.

In both religious and secular Buddhism, the human condition is subjected to subtle or not so subtle condemnation. Religious Buddhism will have you prostrate in front of an altar. Secular Buddhism will send you on an eight-week stress-reduction program. One will have you accumulate merit in a make-believe karmic bank account in view of more favorable incarnations in the future. The other will encourage you to give up powerful emotions and set the goal of tranquility, leaving your very humanity at the door before entering the newly sterilized temple of 'mindful living.'

Bad Life

The resolve (the unexplained and compelling decision) to enter the stream, to bathe in the river of living-and-dying, to accept its inescapable route to the ocean thrusts me beyond the artificial confines of a self-bound existence lived on the riverbank. The resolution is inexorably linked to and echoed by the wide world. It is a decisive act: I decide that I want to remember. I decide to not forget. I take to heart the exhortation 'never forget.'

'Never forget!'—with added exclamation mark—is, of course, Auschwitz's powerful memento, running parallel, if we allow for Adorno's (2005) sombre insight, with the impossibility of poetry after the Nazi camps but also, one is compelled to add, after Amritsar, after Sabra and Shatila, after the Armenian genocide—the list could go on. This wider (unorthodox, yet necessary) remembrance (mindfulness) travels way beyond the narcissism of personal liberation, the self-absorbing dream of individual psychological integration. This is because the notion of a 'good life' surrounded by 'bad life' is futile (Butler, 2012).

In Praise of Reverie

Alongside our emotions, feelings, and the rich and chaotic array comprising of what Marcel Proust (1982) called *upheavals of thought*, another aspect of human experience chastised by a reductive understanding of mindfulness is the natural human tendency for reverie.

To cultivate the mind of awakening through everyday meditative practice—both on and off the cushion—is, of course, a *conscious* resolve, in itself remarkable if one takes into account our tendency to shy away from too much reality. Nonetheless, excessive reliance on the conscious mind is at variance with an embodied dharma practice and more attuned to the Promethean craving of the self to appropriate an organismic field of experience. This is also the stance of positivist psychology, currently dominant and leaning towards "hypertrophied consciousness" (Bollas, 2007: 81).

What unfolds in dharma practice is beyond the reach of the conscious mind. Conscious resolve is needed in order to summon up the aspiration to practice the Buddhadharma. If this were all, however, it would betray a narrowly-conceived subjectivism and a naïve reliance on 'willpower.' Questioning the powers of the conscious mind does not mean advocating a mystical dissolution of the mind. Either position, Dōgen tells us, is a copout. For Dōgen (2002) the very nature of the resolve, of what he calls the 'thought of awakening' (*bodaishin*), is unfathomable:

> [*Bodaishin*] does not exist independently or rise suddenly now in a vacuum. It is neither one nor many, neither spontaneous nor accomplished. [This mind] is not all-pervasive throughout the entire world... Despite all this, the arising of the thought of enlightenment occurs where cosmic resonance presents itself. It is neither furnished by the Buddhas and the bodhisattvas, nor is it one's own effort. Because the thought of enlightenment is awakened through cosmic resonance, it is not natural" (Kim, 1975: 156).

The will of the conscious mind may *ignite* a process, the essential components of which are embedded in personal and social conditions, and augmented by infinite resonance. All of the above are ingenious conceptual efforts on Dōgen's part, pointing to the indefinable and ambivalent nature of *thusness*.

Dharma practice (and dharma *education*) invites us to be a 'person of thusness' (*immonin*), one of Dōgen's favorite phrases. The journey of the person of thusness begins and ends in ambivalence, residing, after all negations have been uttered, in what Dōgen calls *kannō dōkō* or "endless reverberation" (Hisamatsu, 1971: 9). Dharma practice is not only subtle; it is, according to Dōgen, *imperceptible* (Kim, 1975). The 'work' goes on undetected by the conscious mind.

The above will sound familiar to psychotherapists who, counter to the zeitgeist's "embarrassing romancing of consciousness" (Bollas, 2007: 81) and its demands for "evisceration of the work with unconscious experience" (ibid), are not prepared to readily accept the current dismissal of the unconscious. The popularity currently enjoyed by 'mindfulness meditation' and the way in which it is applied to mental health settings might be due to the Promethean emphasis, in our day and age (Rose and Rose, 2013), on the powers of the conscious mind and the reluctance to accept what Joyce McDougall, echoing Freud, calls the *unknowable* (McDougall and Dalai Lama, 1998).

This dominant cultural bias is, perhaps, reflected in the way in which dharma teachings are currently apprehended: favoring *manifest* over *latent* states of consciousness, and relegating the latter to the purgatorial locus of obstructions (*āvaraṇa* in Sanskrit), afflictions (*kleśa*), and imprints (*vāsanā* or, in the language of Western psychology, phylogenetic and transgenerational inheritance). This is, in many ways, parallel to the predominant reading of the unconscious as *Id* in contemporary psychology culture and the concomitant bypassing of its creative and healing possibilities. A worrying tendency, arguably gaining ascendancy at present in the field of mental health, would all too happily relegate the unconscious to the museum of outmoded curiosities in the name of 'progress.'

Flowers of Space

This brings us to another significant point, examined with great subtlety by Dōgen. It concerns the imaginings, daydreaming, associations, thoughts, and feelings—the strange unending procession of dappled things, of things counter, original, spare, and strange emerging in the mind-screen of the meditator. In Dōgen's thirteenth-century Japan these were deemed, disparagingly, as *kuge*, 'flowers in the sky'—fickle diversions from the meditator's serious task. This type of evaluation is comparable, perhaps, to how mindfulness writers are fond of chastising "ruminations" (Martin and Tesser, 1996; Bishop, et al., 2011) said to be playing "a central role in exacerbating negative affect" (Bishop et al., 2011: 236), with the latter usually described as clinging to the past and pining for or worrying about the future. Typically, this is followed in mindfulness literature by exhortations to calm the mind and dwell in the 'here and now.'

Yet the imperative to quieten the mind through the use of a meditative technique may be also seen as a rather despotic attempt to silence the *psyche*, instead of being more humbly receptive to its assorted manifestations. I would like to suggest that this injunction violates the first Buddhist precept: refraining from taking life. It could be argued that the suppression of any emergent phenomenon equally violates the precept. Suppressing what spontaneously arises is different from embracing, experiencing fully, and *then* letting go. Left to their own devices, emergent phenomena vanish in the same spacious atmosphere in which they came into view.

Too single-minded an emphasis on the powers of the conscious mind fails to appreciate the subtlety and complexities of human experience. In his discourse 'This mind itself is Buddha' (*Sokushin-zebutsu*), Dōgen gave a new twist to the meaning of 'flowers in the sky': he re-translated *kuge* as 'flowers of space', phenomena to be embraced and appreciated by the mind's thusness (*shinshō*), instead of being hurriedly and nervously rejected as distractions in a practice erroneously identified with quietism. It would be naïve, Dōgen says, to identify Buddha solely with the discriminating activities of the mind.

The Unconscious Revisited

What begins to emerge and gain momentum from various sources (Bollas, 2007; Ryan, 2007; Panksepp, 2008; Schore and Schore, 2008; Schore, 2012) is that no successful therapy can take place without a subtle level of unconscious communication between client and therapist. The language in which this is expressed varies according to the theoretical orientation. Some will speak of right brain to right brain communication, essential in accessing psychic regions obfuscated by trauma. Others will report on the depth of relating and healing that can take place in moments of unbiased, uncluttered expression. Others still may emphasize the felt sense and the quality of presence, the shared humanity and vulnerability opening new vistas in the therapeutic landscape. Like fingers pointing to the proverbial moon, these reports testify of an unfathomable component playing a crucial role in therapeutic work.

One must resist, however, the urge to brand these dimensions as 'spiritual' or 'transpersonal', for these translations are too literal and close to hijacking an experience that remains—if one cares about intellectual integrity—*unfathomable*. To locate them within the unconscious seems less of a copout, provided the term is not reified, that is, not understood as a 'thing'—retrieved from the mechanistic clutches of orthodox psychoanalysis and realigned with more inspired evocations.

To maintain the notion of an unconscious is a necessary downsizing of the self's labor-intensive claims for exclusive sovereignty over the vast domain of experience and the different layers of inter- and intra-psychic processes. Conversely, to maintain and reinforce the conscious mind is forfeiting psyche in favor of a limited self-construct—essentially an act of *hubris*.

Imperceptible Mutual Assistance

Meditation is a communal act. When sitting together in zazen, Dōgen says, an astonishing thing takes place, unaided and undetected. He calls it *imperceptible mutual assistance* (Kim, 1975). Nothing is said; little is perceived by the conscious mind. Nonetheless, this subtle process takes a life of its own. Provisionally united by a common yet paradoxical (i.e., not goal-oriented) aspiration, we help each other by sitting together in silence.

Often, during an intensive silent meditation retreat, participants feel that a subtle communication is being established. As days unfold, I may feel as if I am strangely getting to know someone intimately, even though not a single word has been exchanged between us. Then, on the last day, with the silence broken, speaking to those very same people over breakfast, I may find that the image I had built of them is contradicted, at times considerably so. Typically, I find myself thinking: 'The image of this person assembled in my own mind was a mere assortment of erroneous impressions, projections, and biases. *This* man or woman sitting opposite me and speaking to me right now is surely the *real* person.'

The above conclusion sounds true enough, yet nowadays I feel less certain as I realize that several things are going on at the same time in perception and communication. The majority of these are not registered by the conscious mind. It would seem that more subtle, unconscious communication takes place unheeded.

Mindfulness and Double-entry Bookkeeping

To conceive of *individual* liberation (or at least of greater freedom from distress) within a socio-political context that is far from liberated only reinforces the notion of the individual as an isolated body–mind unit. It confirms a misleading notion of meditation practice as personal salvation. What is more, by attempting to sever the indissoluble link between individual and societal malaise, it corroborates the view of contemplative practices as opiates, as ways to divert one's attention from historical and political contingencies in order to pursue a path of private deliverance. It also de-contextualizes meditation: for centuries Buddhist meditation has been practiced *communally*, embedded as it was in a cultural and religious milieu.

I am not advocating the preservation of the cultural and ritualistic trappings inevitably inhabited by the dharma in its nomadic journeying through centuries and continents, but instead defending the quintessentially *collective* aspect of meditation practice. A *private* and *technical* conception of dharma practice reflects the notion of a privatized religion which, alongside double-entry bookkeeping, heralded the birth of capitalism and the Protestant worldview.

McMindfulness

I sympathize with the optimism and ambitious claims of much contemporary neuroscience and of similar positivist perspectives, to which mindfulness belongs. Purpose and enthusiasm drive science forward; yet the implicit or explicit message often following positivist assertions is that it will be only a matter of time until the complexities of the psyche will be unravelled and the dilemmas of the human condition explained and resolved.

I feel deeply grateful to 'American Buddhism' and I don't forget that several outstanding teachers first came to the West via North America, where the dharma found fertile soil and loyal support. My own initial tentative steps were inspired by the American beat poets. Yet my fundamental education was steeped, alongside the paradoxical teachings of Zen, in the pessimism of the European philosophical tradition—which perhaps goes to explain why in less charitable moments I perceive the mindfulness phenomenon as the cultural artefact of American naïveté and American bravado—as a very American take on the dharma. Some writers (Purser and Loy, 2013) have similarly referred to "McMindfulness", offering "a universal panacea for resolving almost every area of daily concern."

At the heart of the European philosophical tradition are the hermeneutics of suspicion and the cultivation of perplexity. This point is hardly new or particularly shattering: Nietzsche questioned the supposedly noble claims of conventional morality, Marx critiqued the inbuilt iniquity of the social order, and Freud unveiled the complexities and dark corners of psyche. It took centuries of philosophical and historical tussle and strife to reach the flowering of ingenious doubt presented by these three great thinkers. Encompassed within the hermeneutics of suspicion are major developments of thought across many centuries, a vast canon that continues to grow and ramify. Embedded within the European canon are metaphysics, as well as a *critique* of metaphysics. An articulate critical assessment of metaphysics can only take place when elaborated systems of metaphysics have been developed. Hence, Greek culture gave us Plato *and* Heraclitus, Aristotle *and* Pyrrho. For every architect of metaphysics, an equally ingenious dismantler of certainty came along. There is a Kierkegaard for every Hegel, an Adorno for every Heidegger, and so forth. What's more, each extensive system of thought has its own inbuilt demise: this is one of the meanings of Jacques Derrida's (1974, 1978) *deconstruction*. It would be a naïve philosophy indeed that unquestionably believed in its own solidity and consistency.

I am not for a moment claiming that Europe is the privileged locus of such way of philosophizing. The very notion of 'Europe' is spurious: not only that Europe has deep roots in the East and the Middle East (Said, 1979), but the flowering of European culture is itself the product of exiles (Adorno, 2005; Bazzano, 2006, 2012), rather than the straightforward expression of an imaginary European identity. Moreover, much of European thought has been revitalized over the last few decades in America, whilst arguably stagnating and fossilizing in European academia. A question some writers ask (Hartman, 1982; Vendler, 1988) is whether a restricted canon may engender narrow-minded views. They ask whether being disconnected from the distant past or, as Wallace Stevens says (Vendler, 1988), not having within one's field of vision the vivid and mysterious sight of a Grecian urn might result in holding a strange mix of arrogance and naïveté.

Which is a rather roundabout way of asking: Is mindfulness in its current manifestation an essentially American phenomenon? And what would happen if it were more fully affected by the best European counter-tradition?

References

Adorno, T. (2005) *Minima Moralia: Reflections on Damaged Life* (London: Verso).

Batchelor, S. (1997) *Buddhism without Beliefs: A Contemporary Guide to Awakening* (London: Bloomsbury).

Bazzano, M. (ed.) (2002) *Zen Poems* (London: MQP).

Bazzano, M. (2006) *Buddha is Dead: Nietzsche and the Dawn of European Zen* (Brighton and Portland, OR: Sussex Academic Press).

Bazzano, M. (2011) 'Empathy for the Devil: The Daimonic in Therapy. A Tribute to Jean Genet', *Journal of the Society of Existential Analysis*, 22(1), 150–9.

Bazzano, M. (2012) *Spectre of the Stranger: Towards a Phenomenology of Hospitality* (Brighton and Portland, OR: Sussex Academic Press).

Bazzano, M. (2013a) 'The Buddha Delusion', *Self & Society*, 41(1), 55–60.

Bazzano, M. (2013b) 'In Praise of Stress Induction: Mindfulness Revisited', *European Journal of Psychotherapy and Counselling*, 15(2), 174–85.

Bazzano, M. (2013c) 'Back to the Future: From Behaviourism and Cognitive Psychology to Motivation and Emotion', *Self & Society*, 40, 32–5.

Bishop, S.R., Lau, M. and Shapiro, S. (2011) 'Mindfulness: a Proposed Operational Definition', *Contemporary Buddhism*, 12(1), 230–41.

Bollas, C. (1987) *Forces of Destiny* (London: Free Association Books).

Bollas, C. (2007) *The Freudian Moment* (London: Karnac).

Butler, J. (2012) 'Can One Lead a Good Life in a Bad Life? Adorno Prize Lecture 11 September 2012 Frankfurt', *Radical Philosophy*, 176, 9–18.

Chöpel, G. (2009) *In the Forest of Faded Wisdom: 104 poems by Gendun Chöpel*, edited and translated by D.S. Lopez Jr (Chicago, IL: Chicago University Press).

Derrida, J. (1974) *Of Grammatology* (Baltimore, MD: The Johns Hopkins University Press).

Derrida, J. (1978) *Writing and Difference* (Chicago, IL: University of Chicago).

Dōgen (2002) *The Heart of Dōgen's Shōbōgenzō*, translated and annotated by N. Waddell and M. Abe (Albany, NY: State University of New York).

Freud, S. (1990) *Beyond the Pleasure Principle* (New York: W.W. Norton & Company).

Hartman, G. (1982) *Criticism in the Wilderness: the Study of Literature Today* (London: Yale University Press).

Hillman, J. (1992) *Re-visioning Psychology* (New York: Harper Perennial).

Hisamatsu, S. (1971) *Zen and the Fine Arts* (Tokyo: Kodansha International).

Jung, C. G. (1962) *Commentary on the Secret of the Golden Flower* (New York: Mariner).

Kim, H. J. (1975) *Dōgen, Mystical Realist* (Tucson, AZ: University of Arizona Press).

McDougall, J. and Dalai Lama (1998) 'Is There an Unconscious in Buddhist Teaching? A Conversation Between Joyce McDougall and His Holiness the Dalai Lama', in Molino, A. (ed.) *The Couch and the Tree*, pp. 265–75 (New York: North Point Press).

Madison, G. B. (1981) *The Phenomenology of Merleau-Ponty* (Athens, OH: Ohio University Press).

Maezumi, T. (2001) *Appreciate your Life: the Essence of Zen Practice* (Boston, MA: Shambala).

Martin, L. and Tesser, A. (1996) 'Some Ruminative Thoughts', in Wyer, R. S. (ed.) *Advances in Social Cognition*, vol. 9, pp. 1–48 (Hillsdale, NJ: Lawrence Erlbaum).

May, R. (1969) *Love and Will* (New York: Norton).

Merleau-Ponty, M. (1964) *The Primacy of Perception and Other Essays* (Evanston, IL: Northwestern University Press).

Moreira, V. (2012) 'From Person-centered to Humanistic-phenomenological Psychotherapy: The Contribution of Merleau-Ponty to Carl Rogers's Thought', *Person-Centered and Experiential Psychotherapies,* 11(1), 48–63.

Panksepp, J. (2008) 'The Power of the Word may Reside in the Power of Affect', *Integrative Psychological and Behavioral Science,* 42, 47–55.

Proust, M. (1982) *Remembrance of Things Past,* 3 vols, translated by C.K. Scott Moncrieff and T. Kilmartin (New York: Vintage Press).

Purser, R. and Loy, D. (2013) 'Beyond McMindfulness', available at: http://www.huffingtonpost.com/ron-purser/beyondmcmindfulness_b_3519289.html?goback=.gde_3703348_member_258283471 (accessed 10 July 2013).

Rose, H. and Rose, S. (2013) *Genes, Cells and Brains: the Promethean Promises of the New Biology* (London: Verso).

Ryan, R.M. (2007) 'A New Look and Approach for Two Re-emerging Fields', *Motivation and Emotion,* 31, 1–3.

Said, E. (1979) *Orientalism* (New York: Vintage).

Schore, A. N. (2012) *The Science of the Art of Psychotherapy* (New York: Norton).

Schore J. R. and Schore A. N. (2008) 'Modern Attachment Theory: The Central Role of Affect Regulation in Development and Treatment', *Clinical Social Work Journal,* 36, 9–20.

Spinelli, E. (2007) *Practising Existential Psychotherapy: The Relational World* (London: SAGE).

Thera, N (1973) *The Heart of Buddhist Mindfulness* (New York: Samuel Weiser).

Vendler, H. (1988) *The Music of what Happens* (Cambridge, MA: Harvard University Press).

Virgil, P. M. (2013) 'Georgics', Book IV, verses 562–56, available at: http://www.theoi.com/Text/VirgilGeorgics1.html (accessed 22 October 2013).

Zupancic, A. (2012) 'Alenka Zupancic on Bio-morality', available at: http://philosophy.atmhs.com/2012/02/25/alenka-zupancic-on-bio-morality (accessed 10 July 2013).

Part II

Beyond Personal Liberation: Mindfulness, Society, and Clinical Practice

6
How Social is Your Mindfulness?
Towards a Mindful Sex and Relationship Therapy
Meg Barker

Introduction

The proliferation and popularity of mindfulness therapies in recent years has enabled many people to access Buddhist theories and practices that are helpful in addressing distress. However, most of the therapies that have been developed so far seem to adopt the dualistic modern Western way of understanding experience rather than taking seriously the non-dualistic approach within which Buddhist understandings are embedded. In this chapter I argue that a biopsychosocial perspective is more in keeping with the theoretical foundations of mindfulness, while also being in line with more recent Western theories. Such a perspective requires giving serious attention to the social context in which we struggle, which has been neglected by the internal focus of much psychotherapy. Specifically, we need to engage with the self-monitoring culture of acquisition and avoidance that currently pervades Western society. I refer to such an approach as 'social mindfulness' to distinguish it from those mindful approaches that engage less explicitly with the social.

This chapter illustrates these points with the example of sex and relationship therapies. So far, the focus of mindfulness in these areas has been on applying techniques to complement conventional therapies which, broadly speaking, aim at enabling couples to have conventional sex and to stay together in romantic relationships (Barker, 2013a). If sex and relationship therapies are to be mindful, then they need to go beyond this and critically examine the sociocultural understandings of sex and relationships that people draw upon. In particular, they need to address the approach/avoidance patterns that are encouraged, for example, by mainstream media and many psychiatric, psychological, and psychotherapeutic understandings of sex and relationships. We need to ask what kinds of sex and relationships people are trying to have and why, rather than accepting these as taken-for-granted. Long term, a more appropriate aim for mindful sex and relationship therapy (in terms of both individual suffering and the wider world) would be to help people to "swim against the stream" (Batchelor, 2010: 125) of problematic social norms and cultural assumptions, rather than continuing to work towards enabling them to fit these.

I write as somebody who has engaged with mindfulness in three ways. First, I have been reading Western Buddhist authors such as Stephen Batchelor (1997, 2010), Martine Batchelor (2001), and Pema Chödrön (1994, 2001) for the last two decades, and trying to apply their ideas and practices to my own daily life. Second, I have engaged with Buddhist ideas and practices academically, considering what they have to offer methodologically and theoretically in terms of the ways in which we study and understand human experience (see Stanley et al., in press). And, third, I have attempted to integrate Buddhist theory and practice into my own therapeutic work, training, and writing, which involves bringing it into dialogue with existential–humanistic and social constructionist perspectives. This has culminated recently in my own book, which explores current versions of mindfulness and sets out a proposal for a more critically informed and socially engaged mindful therapy (Barker, 2013b), as well as general audience writings that explore romantic relationships from a mindful perspective (Barker, 2013c).

I am aware of the gaps in my own knowledge and experience given that I am not, by any means, a Buddhist scholar. Nor, despite my background in psychology, do I have the in-depth knowledge of cognitive–behavioural psychology or neuroscience that many contributors to these debates have. Therefore, I apologise in advance for the necessary oversimplifications in the following arguments. I recognise, for example, that some Western authors on mindfulness have engaged with social context and with the tensions that I explore here (e.g., see Williams and Kabat-Zinn, 2011), although such engagements do not always filter down to mindfulness practices in settings that have historically employed medical and/or cognitive–behavioural therapies (CBT), which are what I am generally speaking of when I refer to 'Western mindfulness.' Additionally, I simply cannot do justice here to the diversity present in the vast array of forms of Buddhism that exist now and historically when I speak of 'Buddhist philosophies.' Finally, I am aware of the range of 'Western psychotherapies' that—to a greater or lesser extent—critically engage with the project of diagnosing and treating disorders.

Western Therapeutic Approaches to Suffering

Broadly speaking, Western psychotherapy, psychology, and psychiatry regard human distress as a problem that requires treatment. The focus of the endeavour for the last century or more has been on determining the different kinds of distress that people experience; categorising these as disorders, abnormalities, or mental illnesses; locating their cause (e.g., in their neurochemistry and/or thought processes); and developing physical and psychological treatments with the aim of curing the problems and ameliorating the distress. So, for example, a cluster of symptoms whereby a person has low mood, feels tired, and thinks badly of themselves may be classified as 'depression', located in their levels of serotonin and/or tendency towards negative self-attributions, and treated with 'anti-depressants' and/or CBT (Pilgrim, 2010).

Such an approach—echoed in wider societal understandings of mental health (Barker, 2011a)—involves fixing the person *as* their problem: it is something that they *are* or something that they *have* as an internal aspect of who they are, like a personality trait or other individual characteristics. So we divide people into the emotionally, psychologically, or mentally well and unwell, and consider them as *being* depressed, psychotic, or personality disordered, or as *having* anxiety, a paraphilia, or a sexual dysfunction.

Such categorising relates to the ways in which human distress is understood by such approaches to mental health: generally it is located within the person and the focus is upon internal (biological and/or psychological) causes. Thus, the Western scientific model of cause–effect relationships is applied to human experience, as it is assumed that each emotional state or behaviour will have an identifiable cause, probably in internal cognitive processes. This is a dualistic approach that regards causes and effects, minds and bodies, thoughts and behaviours, emotions and cognitions, and individuals and other individuals as separable and as having the capacity to act upon each other in cause–effect relationships.

So, for example, in the arena of sex therapy, a person may come to a psychotherapist or counselling psychologist saying that they are unable to achieve an erection. They will be categorised as having 'erectile dysfunction' and as being sexually disordered. This will be regarded as an effect with an underlying cause: most likely a physiological condition of the blood vessels of the penis, or a psychological issue relating to anxiety around sexual performance. This may be treated with a phosphodiesterase type 5 (PDE5) inhibitor drug and/or CBT to challenge negative automatic thoughts and to reduce anxiety about sex, perhaps through gradually building up to penetration via other forms of physical touch to increase confidence in the ability to sustain an erection.

When it comes to difficulties in a relationship beyond the sexual arena, relationship therapists are less likely to diagnose an individual (although some diagnostic categories, such as personality disorders, do include relationship problems as criteria). More likely it will be the relationship that is viewed as dysfunctional or classed as a 'relationship problem.' The cause of the problem will still be internally located, often within the thought processes of the individuals, but also within the dynamic between the people in the relationship. Thus, there is some sense of people as interconnected, although the couple unit is still treated as relatively separate from the social world in most therapy. The focus of therapy depends upon the therapeutic approach taken, with humanistic, psychodynamic and systemic approaches being as common as CBT in this area. Treatment might involve, for example, shifting the attributions that each member of a couple makes about each other (so that they reverse the tendency to blame good behaviour on external factors and bad behaviour on internal ones), providing communication skills training, or bringing dynamics out into the open (e.g., if one person's nagging tends to result in the other's withdrawal, which results in the first person pushing harder, etc.). There may be some exploration of the background of each person which led to their characters developing in the ways they did.

Western Mindfulness: Perpetuating not Problematising?

Considering the most popular forms of Western mindfulness that have emerged, and reached prominence, in the last two decades, it seems to me that these add some of the key practices and theories of Buddhism to Western psychotherapies, but sometimes fail to engage with the challenges that Buddhist philosophies pose to the popular psychological understandings of human experience and distress outlined above.

These mindfulness therapies most frequently add mindfulness to CBT, an approach rooted in cognitive–experimental psychology with its emphasis on determining causes of human behaviours and focus on the individual human being (e.g., in comparison to the wider social focus of sociology, or cultural studies). We can see the predominance of such an approach in the mindfulness research that has been published to date, after the explosion of interest in this topic a decade or so ago. The vast bulk of this research has concentrated on determining an operational definition of mindfulness; measuring the degree of mindfulness a person has; finding out whether mindfulness therapies are effective at decreasing problems such as depression, stress or pain; and examining how mindfulness practice works in the brain (Cohen, 2010).

Therapeutically, these Western mindfulness approaches involve introducing clients to meditative, and other, practices that cultivate the ability to bring non-judgemental attention to the present moment, rather than constantly evaluating experience and/or becoming distracted by thoughts of the past or the future. However, such techniques are generally introduced as a way of treating specific 'disorders' or 'dysfunctions' (e.g., depression or anxiety) and therefore still involve separating out and addressing different forms of distress that are regarded as something intrinsic to the individual.

The focus of such mindfulness approaches is also internal, as the causes of distress are located in the individual's relationship to their thought processes and/or emotional states. The aim of mindfulness practice is generally to shift habitual mental patterns and change how we relate to experience by developing the capacity to be in the present moment rather than ruminating on the past or focusing upon achieving future goals. It also involves a shift from avoiding experience to approaching it (Segal et al., 2002); from changing things to accepting how they are (Hayes, 2005); and/or from a threat-based approach to a more compassionate approach to experience (Gilbert, 2010). There is little engagement, across the literature on mindfulness, with the *context* in which distress occurs, or critical consideration of the Western psychological/psychotherapeutic ways of understanding humans and their distress that underlie such approaches to mental health.

Returning to sex and relationship therapy then, a Western mindfulness approach to the same issue that we considered above would generally still classify the person as having 'erectile dysfunction' and emphasise the role of psychological factors in causing such problems (after ruling out any underlying physiological problem). However, rather than focusing on reducing anxiety about sex and increasing confidence, it might concentrate more upon tuning in to bodily responses and cultivating the ability to be in the present moment, rather than ruminating over past experiences of poor performance or worrying that it will go wrong this time. Mindfulness exercises such as breathing meditation, paying attention to body sensations, and observing thoughts coming and going without judgement would be added to more conventional education about sexual functioning (e.g., Brotto et al., 2008; Goldmeier and Mears, 2010). Therapy might also involve challenging of negative thinking patterns and sexual arousal exercises, and the client would be encouraged to approach the anxiety-provoking situation rather than avoid it (Brotto and Barker, 2013).

So far, Western mindfulness approaches have been applied less to relationship therapy than to sex therapy. However, work that has been conducted in this area is similar to that in the area of sexual dysfunction in that it generally retains conventional understandings of relationship problems, while adding on mindfulness techniques as a way of addressing these. For example, Carson et al. base their application of mindfulness to relationship therapy on the argument that 'healthy individual functioning is important to successful marriages' (2004: 472). This retains the focus on internal individual causes of problems—or their lack—not to mention equating relationships with marriage and taking for granted what it means for one to be successful. In their programme, standard Western mindfulness techniques and explanations were added on to a pre-existing relationship course that included the kinds of skills instruction and couple exercises common to relationship therapy.

Social Mindfulness

I will now outline a social mindfulness perspective as a possible alternative to the most popular forms of Western mindfulness sketched above, before applying this in detail to sex and relationships in the remainder of the chapter.

Social mindfulness has emerged in the last few years in the UK out of a critique of the ways in which Western psychotherapy and psychology has engaged with Buddhist philosophy to date (Stanley, 2012). The alternative form of social mindfulness put forward attempts to do two things differently:

1. To engage more fully with the Buddhist philosophies within which mindfulness was initially embedded, and with current Buddhist thought and practice, integrating the social aspects of experience more fully than current Western mindfulness.
2. To bring Buddhist theories and practices into dialogue with those Western approaches that explicitly engage with the social level of existence—sociology, cultural theory, existential philosophy, and

critical psychology. This involves drawing upon the work of writers such as de Beauvoir, Foucault, Butler, and Deleuze, who emphasise the embodied nature of experience and the role of social power in the construction of identity.

Table 6.1 outlines the different conceptualisations of social mindfulness: of distress; of human beings; of the causes of experience, including distress; and of the appropriate way of therapeutically engaging with distress. Each of these points will be developed in the remainder of this section.

Broadly speaking, Western mindfulness adds a form of mindfulness onto existing Western psychotherapy rather than allowing mindfulness—and its underlying philosophy—into a dialogue that might challenge the assumptions implicit within Western psychological and therapeutic approaches. Perhaps the most obvious tension here is the fact that Western therapies view human distress as something to be treated and eradicated—a problem to be fixed—while Buddhist philosophies generally regard distress of various kinds as an inevitable

Table 6.1 Key differences between popular Western mindfulness approaches and the social mindfulness approach.

	Western mindfulness approaches	Social mindfulness approaches
Distress	A problem to be treated and eradicated, albeit sometimes in different ways to standard psychotherapy	Inevitable and therefore to be embraced as part of life
Human beings	Separate individuals who may be ordered/disordered, healthy/ill, normal/abnormal	Interconnected beings, inseparable from each other and the world they occupy
Cause of experiences	Internal biological and/or psychological factors	No causes but rather a constant co-arising of a complex interaction of biopsychosocial processes
Cause of distress	Habitual ways of relating to thoughts, feelings, and sensations	Craving for things to be otherwise, self-monitoring based on societal norms
Therapy	Techniques in which we non-judgementally attend to the present moment	Critical engagement with the way discourses operate through us via mindful practices and reflection

part of being human. Buddhist mindfulness practices are part of the path towards accepting that our suffering is rooted in our very attempts to avoid and eradicate distress. We practice mindfulness in order to observe our habitual tendency to try to get all of the things we want and to avoid or get rid of all of the things that we don't want. In slowing down and observing such cravings at an everyday level, we can see how our suffering is rooted within them.

Western mindfulness approaches do engage, to some extent, with these understandings, for example by advising approaching difficult experiences such as fear and anxiety, rather than avoiding them (Crane, 2009), and by cultivating the capacity to accept experience as it is rather than engaging in goal-directed attempts to change it (Flaxman et al., 2011). However, there is little engagement with the conflict inherent in the fact that this is often still done in the name of treating 'disorders, such as depression and anxiety, sexual 'dysfunctions', or relationship 'problems.' We remain at risk of endeavouring to escape or avoid distress rather than taking seriously the inevitability of suffering in life and addressing how we engage with this.

For this reason—and because of the concentration on finding internal causes of suffering—the client in Western mindfulness therapy may well still feel as though they are lacking or flawed in some way *because* they are struggling. Western therapy, from a Buddhist perspective, could be regarded as implicated in suffering because it reinforces and perpetuates the idea that struggling is pathological, rather than normal, and that it can be eradicated through the therapeutic process, or through becoming mindful enough. Despite its emphasis on *being* rather than *doing*, some forms of Western mindfulness are in danger of sneaking back in the goal of removing all pain from life (see Magid, 2008). They may well contribute to client's self-blame and suffering when mindfulness—just like everything else they have tried—fails to accomplish the total eradication of pain.

If we consider the wider sociocultural context in which Western psychotherapy has developed, and in which Western mindfulness has been embraced, these paradoxes become more explicable. Psychotherapy emerged in the 'Panopticonic' society that resulted from industrialisation, secularism, individualism, and consumer capitalism (Foucault, 1975). As in the perfect Panopticon prison, where prisoners know that they may be watched by the guard at any time and therefore start to police their own behaviour, modern society encourages people to continuously monitor and police themselves and others. Via mainstream media and the babble of everyday conversation, a sense of anxiety

is created about things we lack (e.g., beauty, youth, love, or pleasure). We are encouraged to compare our individual, atomised selves
against (idealised) others and to find ourselves wanting (Barker, 2013c).
We are then required to buy products, read magazines, watch televi-
sion programmes, and engage in various forms of self-improvement in
an attempt to fix ourselves. This is doomed to failure because there will
always be further lacks to uncover as we continue to scrutinise ourselves,
our bodies, our relationships, and our lives for the ways in which they
are wanting (Gergen, 2000).

Psychotherapy can be seen as part of the Panopticon, encouraging us
to attend to our 'neuroses' or 'negative thoughts', and to engage in an
endless project of self-perfection in a desperate attempt to be 'normal':
to fix the disorders and dysfunctions that psychotherapy told us that we
had in the first place (Kutchins and Kirk, 1997). Given the lack of disclo-
sure by the psychotherapist, it is easy for the client to assume that the
therapist, unlike the client, is, in comparison, another normal person
(Barker et al., 2010).

Given this, it is all too easy for mindfulness to simply become the
new way in which we are flawed: not mindful enough, or not happy in
the ways in which the positive psychology movement suggests that we
would be if we were more mindful. Similarly, it is easy for meditation
and other practices to become the latest commodity (Carrette and King,
2005), and a stick to beat ourselves with as we realise that we are not
doing it enough, or properly, or whatever we would need to be doing in
order to finally stop struggling (Chödrön, 1994).

The Western mindfulness emphasis on paying non-judgemental
attention to the present moment as an internal individual solution
to psychological difficulties risks missing the wider social context in
which such difficulties emerge. This is true of situations of alienation,
stigmatisation, and oppression, which statistics on different levels of
diagnosis across gender, race, sexuality, and so on, clearly implicate
in distress (Barker et al., 2010). It is also true of the wider Western
craving culture that encourages us to relate to other people and the
world via attachment/aversion—precisely what, according to Buddhism,
exacerbates suffering (Barker, 2013b).

Buddhist philosophy is, on the whole, non-dualistic. This is at variance with the models of human being inherent in most psychological
therapies, and in current Western understanding more broadly, which,
as we have seen, separate out minds and bodies, thoughts and feelings, and self and other. The Panopticonic view, which regards us as
atomised beings with individual identities to be monitored, compared

against others, and improved, is alien to much Buddhist philosophy as I understand it (from my reading of the work of Buddhist scholars such as Batchelor (1997), Bazzano (2012), and those who contributed to the collection by Williams and Kabat-Zinn (2011)). If engaged with fully, this would point to a potentially highly valuable way of addressing suffering: by questioning the notion of static, separate, and bounded individuals who can be evaluated in such ways, and emphasising instead the interconnectedness and intersubjectivity inherent in being-in-the-world-with-others (Nhat Hanh, 1975; Gergen, 2009).

Non-dualistic Buddhist philosophy is consistent with more recent Western critical theory about health, which stresses that we are embodied beings (not separate minds and bodies) and that all experience is simultaneously biopsychosocial, and that it would be impossible to tease these elements apart (Fox, 2012). We are embodied biological beings *and* psychological experiencers *and* inextricably *situated* in our social worlds. As Stephen Batchelor explains:

> We have been created, moulded, formed by a bewildering matrix of contingencies that have preceded us. From the patterning of the DNA derived from our parents to the firing of the hundred billion neurons in our brains to the cultural and historical conditioning of the twentieth [now twenty-first] century to the education and upbringing given us to all the experience we have ever had and choices we have ever made: these have conspired to configure the unique trajectory that culminates in this present moment (1997:82).

This 'bewildering matrix' renders nonsensical simplistic splits like mind/body, nature/nurture, or hard-wired/chosen behaviours. It also challenges the common psychological assumption of cause–effect relationships, which are overly simplistic when it comes to open systems like human beings. There are moves in Western theory and science away from such simplistic understandings that resonate with Buddhist perspectives (e.g., see Varela et al., 1991, and Fox, 2012), while much mainstream psychological and psychotherapeutic work (including much of the research on mindfulness) seems to retain such assumptions.

A Socially Mindful Sex Therapy

What might a social mindfulness therapeutic approach to sex and relationships look like? Conventional sex therapy diagnoses people as having 'sexual dysfunctions', regarded as problems that require fixing by determining their physiological and/or psychological causes, and addressing these. Thus far, the research literature arguing for the involvement of mindfulness in sex therapy has focused on the potential of mindfulness practices to achieve the same aims as conventional sex therapy (sexual desire, lasting erections, penetration, and orgasm) (Suttie, 2013). Some have pointed out the commonalities between mindfulness and the sex therapy staple of sensate focus whereby the emphasis is taken off genital sex and partners attempt to be present to all sensations they are experiencing (Goldmeier and Mears, 2010). However, such gradation techniques often sneak back in an overall goal of penis-in-vagina penetration and/or orgasm, and the implicit assumptions inherent that this is what constitutes 'good' or 'proper' sex (Barker, 2011b). Some have even suggested that mindfulness could enable people to have penis-in-vagina sex when they are not aroused, or when finding it painful, owing to an openness to all sensations, which is part of why mindfulness is a helpful practice for chronic pain (see Brotto and Barker, 2013).

Such an approach is problematic in both its insistence on a certain form of sex and its failure to understand the embodied nature of human beings. More existential–humanistic therapists have argued that we need to listen to bodies that are refusing to be penetrated, to become erect, or to orgasm, as there may well be good reasons for this (Barker and Langdridge, in press). For example, young women with vaginismus are often involved in some degree of self-objectification and trying to be what others want them to be. The body's refusal to be penetrated could thus be regarded as useful and explicable, and attempts to achieve penetration through gradual insertion of thicker dilators (classic sex therapy) or mindful practice to deal with pain, both seem deeply problematic in this light (Barker, 2011c). Similarly, penises that fail to become erect or to ejaculate may be communicating important things about the pressures around masculinity, the relationship the person is in, or wider anxieties about performance or success (Kleinplatz, 2004). Given the non-dualistic philosophy in which mindfulness is embedded, a holistic biopsychosocial form of therapeutic engagement that took account of these psychosocial meanings would seem to be more appropriate.

Any mindful sex therapy that sneaks in the aim of a particular kind of sex risks being goal-oriented, rather than pleasure/experience-oriented. Social theorists in this area have pointed out the heteronormativity and gender bias involved in what is considered to be the appropriate goal of sex therapy, with its insistence on erect penises reaching orgasm through penetration of vaginas (Barker, 2011b). Such an approach is in contradiction with mindfulness approaches that are aware of the problems inherent in a goal focus that create gaps between where we are and where we want to be (Crane, 2009).

Mindful sex therapy needs to take seriously the implications of—and reasons for—the mindful emphasis on being present to experience, and on shifting from a goal-oriented 'doing' mode to a 'being' mode. It is not enough to teach mindful practices as an addition to conventional goal-directed therapy.

A more social form of mindful sex therapy would take the present focus of mindfulness, not as a way of moving towards standard sexual goals, but rather as a starting point for critical engagement with the social context in which sexual problems emerge. This might include the constructions of femininity or masculinity mentioned above, the ways in which we are alienated from our bodies, or the current imperative to be sexual in particular ways, and the self-monitoring and judgement that this leads to.

Mindful practice can be employed to invite clients into a phenomenological exploration of their lived experience of sex. Instead of engaging in sex with particular aims, they can begin to bring mindful attention to sex and thus notice what is happening in terms of their sensations, feelings and thoughts during the experience.

One activity that I have found useful is to encourage people to pick a particular kind of sensual, erotic, or sexual experience that they have experienced as both fulfilling and not fulfilling. This could be a sexual practice with another person, masturbation, flirting, receiving a massage, cybersex, or anything else that they would put into this category. People then remember the experiences, in rich detail, through the kind of spacious attention that takes in everything equally, writing a thorough description of both the fulfilling and not fulfilling versions of the experience. Discussion then focuses on the difference between the two versions.

What generally emerges from this comparison is that the differences are akin to the differences between engaging in an experience more or less mindfully (see Barker, 2011d). In the fulfilling experience, people are present rather than worrying about previous experiences or thinking about what is coming next. They generally feel engaged in the flow of what is happening rather than finding themselves distracted. They feel embodied rather than experiencing a separation of body and mind whereby they are evaluating how they look in this position or whether their bodies are responding or performing 'right.'

It is useful to engage in a reflective exploration of what is getting in the way in the non-fulfilling experience and causing those jagged edges that disrupt an easy sense of flow. Often, the main blockage is the babble of monitoring self-talk that the person is engaged in during sex. This is embedded within the social understandings that surround us about what we *should* be doing: the media images of sex we've been bombarded with, the script for 'successful' sex, and the comparisons we make against imagined others.

If our mindful observations of sexual experience do lead to the conclusion that our struggles with sex are interwoven with the social context within which we are embedded, then the therapeutic endeavour becomes a double-pronged approach. First, we attempt to bring a more mindful form of attention to the sex we are having. Second, we critically engage with those social understandings such that we may see them more clearly for what they are and how they operate through us. Through this we may become able to treat these understandings more lightly, rather than becoming attached to them and caught up in their story.

What we likely find through such a critical engagement is that our approach to sex is shot through with craving patterns of attachment and aversion, all of which are reinforced by the world around us (Loy, 2008), including conventional psychological and psychotherapeutic understandings of sex. Both everyday understanding and psychiatric diagnosis divide sex into normal and abnormal, functional and dysfunctional, and place huge importance on 'getting it right.' Therefore, during sex we are likely trying hard to match up to 'good sex' (which happens this often, lasts this long, requires men to naturally know exactly what to do, and results in erection, penetration, and orgasm). Anything without these elements is judged inferior, dysfunctional, or even not sex at all. There is also fear of straying into 'bad sex', which is still pathologised as 'paraphilic' (any kind of excitement at certain sensations or materials, at being watched or watching others, or at mixing sex with pain or power). We are attached to normal, functional, good sex, and attempt to avoid/eradicate abnormal, dysfunctional, bad sex. We walk a fine tightrope between the two as sexual norms and mores shift rapidly, and what constitutes great sex involves straying just far enough into the dangerous, exciting stuff, but not too far (Barker, 2013c).

A Buddhist approach to sex would involve noticing and challenging such internal and social patterns of attachment and aversion that make it nigh on impossible to be present and fulfilled during sex. A more mindful engagement would involve opening to our sexual and other desires, and to the embodied conversation that is happening between partners during sex. This does not mean behaving unethically, given that, in Buddhism, mindfulness is intrinsically linked to compassion and commitment to ethical behaviours. We would attempt to tune in to both our own bodies and desires, and to those of our partner. This would include questioning the current imperative to be sexual—in the narrow way in which this is defined—at all (Richards and Barker, 2013).

We should encourage clients into a full biopsychosocial engagement in sex, considering their lived experience in detail and how it relates to the social understandings around them which operate through them (in their psychological experience of self-monitoring) and play out on and in the bodies of themselves and their partners. Part of this certainly involves engaging in mindful practice. Mindful sex becomes more possible if we cultivate the ability to be present to experience and to notice and attend to all aspects of it in other, less loaded, areas of life such as washing dishes, driving, or sitting. Practices like body scan and walking meditation may well enable us to tune into our bodies better. Here, the aim would be to realise that we are embodied, rather than to trick or force the body into doing what is socially expected of it through practices that enable us to relax more or to handle pain and unpleasurable experience.

More radically still, we may find that such mindful engagement with sex enables us to bring the same qualities of noticing and critical social engagement to other aspects of our lives, and to reach a wider understanding of the ways in which the social operates through us and can be resisted. This is something that I will return to in the conclusion to the chapter.

A Socially Mindful Relationship Therapy

We have seen previously that relationship therapy is generally somewhat less internally-focused than sex therapy owing to it being less mired in diagnostic categories and attending more to the dynamics between the people in a relationship. However, relationship therapy is still generally goal-directed, with the aim of helping couples in distress to resolve their issues and find ways to stay together (Relate, 2013). This aim fits with wider government and cultural contexts that regard divorce, separation, single parenting, and living alone as social ills, and coupledom, monogamy, marriage, and the nuclear family as the 'right' way to relate and to bring up children. There is rarely an exploration, in relationship therapy, of this wider social context in which we experience our romantic relationships, nor of the relatively recent emergence of the romantic partnership, love marriage, and nuclear family compared to the massive diversity of ways of relating that has been present across history, and remains so globally (Barker, 2013c).

For example, being romantic or sexual with more than one person is generally only understood in the context of cheating and infidelity, as an inevitable danger to the couple unit, and something to be avoided or eradicated, rather than recognising the global minority status of monogamy or the diversity of open non-monogamies that exist (Barker and Langdridge, 2010).

Like sex therapy, Western mindful approaches to relationship therapy so far generally retain the goals of resolving issues internal to the couple and enabling them to stay together. They suggest that this could be achieved through mindful practices, for example by facilitating couples to listen to each other, to be more compassionate, and more present to each other. There is little or no critical engagement with what kind of relationship we are aiming for and why, or what makes a 'successful' relationship (e.g., see the concept of the 'mindful couple' put forward by Walser and Westrup, 2008).

The neglect of the current social context is a serious one given that this has a key role in creating relationship distress. As Loy (2008) points out, romantic relationships have become bound up in our personal happiness and fulfilment in recent decades: people look to romantic relationships to reach a permanent state of 'happily-ever-after.' At the same time, people are living longer and are also encouraged to develop and reach their own individual goals in life, with greater gender equality meaning that both people in most couple relationships are focused on being personally fulfilled, as well as having a 'good relationship.'

As with sex, this situation exacerbates the patterns of attachment and aversion to which Buddhist philosophies suggest that we are already so prone (see Batchelor, 2007; Chödrön, 2001). In romantic relationships this means that we devote much time and energy to finding 'The One' perfect person who will complete us and always love us. When imperfections inevitably emerge, we either continue our quest in the form of serial monogamy or secret infidelities where we search for what our current relationship is lacking. Alternatively, we remain monogamously together with that person and collude in presenting an illusion of perfection to everyone else (which perpetuates the myth for them), while privately struggling with failure of the relationship to meet our unrealistic expectations. This may take the form of resigned disillusionment, or cycles of conflict as we fight against perceived flaws or being seen as flawed by the other person. Many people stay in painful and damaging relationships partly owing to the pressure to be in the relationship, or the conviction that they have found the 'right' person and there won't be anybody else for them (Barker, 2013c).

As with sex therapy, social mindfulness can help people to recognise the ways in which such social discourses, scripts, and imagery operate through them. For example, I have found an adapted form of Pema Chödrön's (1994) description of *tonglen* practice to be extremely helpful in noticing the expectations and assumptions around romantic relationships that are in play at times of conflict or disappointment. In this practice we deliberately engage with difficult and painful emotions, rather than avoiding or attempting to escape then. We use these experiences explicitly to connect with the person who we are struggling with in our shared vulnerability.

Through such practices we may become increasingly aware of the ways in which we look to romantic relationships to validate ourselves and to prove that we are okay really. Unfortunately, however good our partners are at this (or we are for our partners), our own secret convictions, from being embedded in self-monitoring culture, that we are really fundamentally lacking in some way, bubble up. We become resentful of our partner for not keeping this at bay; desperate at our own inability to keep the 'bad' sides of ourselves hidden; or angry at our partner for revealing their own imperfections. At such times we easily start to look elsewhere and engage in either/or thinking: they are either perfect and we must stay together or they are imperfect and we must break-up; this is either their fault or it is our fault; we are either the good guy or the bad guy (Barker, 2013c).

Writers such as Chödrön (1994) and Wellwood (1996) offer alternatives to such patterns, which point the way to what a more socially mindful form of relationship therapy might look like. We can slow down and notice, for example, the desire for a partner to be everything to us; either/or thinking about whether we are together/separate; ideas that they belong to us or that we need to fix ourselves in a particular way for them; or the tendency to quantify what we give them and they give us. We can see how experiences of anger, insecurity, and jealousy are shot through with such flickering thoughts and how these, in turn, come from the social milieu we are embedded in: how we have learnt to respond in this way from a million love songs, romantic comedies, magazine articles, and soap operas (Barker, 2013c).

Instead of continuing the pattern of defensively protecting our vulnerabilities and searching for the perfect relationship that will validate us and keep us safe, we can instead open up to communicating and attending to these vulnerabilities. As Wellwood (1996) suggests, relationship therapy can become a process of exploring the ways in which we want our partners to see us, and the ways in which we fear being seen, and embracing the latter as part of us rather than pushing it away.

Such a process necessitates a wider critical consideration of the social context in which we are encouraged to view romantic relationships in such problematic ways, and to develop such impossibly high expectations and restrictive assumptions of what a good relationship looks like. Such critical explorations may also involve questioning why only certain kinds of relationships are socially accepted and encouraged, and others excluded or prohibited to a greater or lesser extent (same-sex romantic relationships; romantic relationships between more than two people; non-romantic relationships, such as close friendships between men, non-sexual relationships, etc.). Instead of seeing the romantic relationship as the only vital relationship in our lives, which requires constant monitoring and evaluation, and seeking therapy if it goes 'wrong', we might shift to viewing ourselves as being in multiple relationships of different kinds, all of which are valuable (Barker et al., in press). This includes relationships with all the other humans with whom we live, work, and connect; with animals; with the world; and with ourselves. Such an approach is less dualistic in relation to self and other than conventional relationship therapy. Under such an understanding, the goals of relationship therapy shift from a scrutiny of the dynamic between us and how it is failing, to an exploration of how wider pressures operate on the relationship. Recognising that we are inevitably in relation with each other may take the pressure off the either/or of 'staying together' or 'breaking up.' We might consider how we can open up to all of the relationships in our lives rather than placing so much emphasis on this particular one.

All of this can move us from a mode of constant inward self-monitoring and self-policing to a more open mode of acceptance of our vulnerabilities and frailties, and of greater engagement with others.

Conclusions

A socially mindful engagement with sex and relationships is non-dualistic because it does not separate out psychological experience from social context, and therefore challenges any entirely *internal* explanation of distress. Such an approach calls upon us and our clients to think critically about the social messages that are operating through us and to start to 'swim against the stream' of our habitual ways of being (Batchelor, 2010). As we have seen, in relation to sex this involves questioning the divisions between 'good' and 'bad' sex commonly accepted and perpetuated by psychiatry, psychology, and psychotherapy. In relation to relationships, this involves questioning the dominant view of romantic relationships. Through a non-dualistic approach to therapy we might find ourselves in a position to better see the role of sociocultural forces and power dynamics in our client's distress. We might be able to better understand the ways in which our own psychologies and therapies are sometimes implicated in exacerbating, rather than ameliorating, suffering.

We need to ask whether it behoves the (socially) mindful therapist to engage on a social, as well as an individual, therapeutic level. My own belief is that we should not simply be applying mindfulness with individuals or groups, but rather we should be raising wider, vital questions in the worlds of therapy and psychology about how sociocultural contexts create conditions of sexual, relational, and other suffering, and how psychotherapy and psychology may be complicit in this in its categories and treatments.

The mindful therapist would also be a social activist, as some have argued the historical Buddha was, whose work would ideally leave both psychotherapy and the wider world irrevocably transformed.

References

Barker, M. (2011a) 'Mental Health Beyond the 1 in 4', available at: http://rewritingtherules.wordpress.com/2011/10/16/mental-health-beyond-the-1-in-4 (accessed 1 February 2013).

Barker, M. (2011b) 'Existential Sex Therapy', *Sexual and Relationship Therapy*, 26(1), 33–47.

Barker, M. (2011c) 'De Beauvoir, Bridget Jones' Pants and Vaginismus', *Existential Analysis*, 22(2), 203–16.

Barker, M. (2011d) 'Mindfulness: It Ain't What you do it's the Way That you do it', available at: http://socialmindfulness.wordpress.com/2011/04/03/mindfulness-it-aint-what-you-do-its-the-way-that-you-do-it/ (accessed 3 February 2013).

Barker, M. (2013a) 'Reflections: Towards a Mindful Sexual and Relationship Therapy', *Sexual & Relationship Therapy*, 28(1–2), 148–52.

Barker, M. (2013b) *Mindful Counselling & Psychotherapy: Practising Mindfully Across Approaches and Issues* (London: SAGE).

Barker, M. (2013c) *Rewriting the Rules: An Integrative Guide to Love, Sex and Relationships* (London: Routledge).

Barker, M. and Langdridge, D. (2010) 'Whatever Happened to Non-monogamies? Critical Reflections on Recent Research and Theory', *Sexualities*, 13(6), 748–72.

Barker, M. and Langdridge, D. (in press) 'Sexuality and Embodiment in Rela-tionships', in Iacovou, S. and Van Deurzen, E. (eds) *Existential Perspectives on Relationship Therapy* (Basingstoke: Palgrave Macmillan).

Barker, M., Vossler, A. and Langdridge, D. (eds) (2010) *Understanding Counselling and Psychotherapy* (London: SAGE).

Barker, M., Heckert, J. and Wilkinson, E. (in press) 'Queering Polyamory: From One Love, to Many, and Back Again', in Sanger, T. and Taylor, Y. (eds) *Intimacies: Relations, Exchanges, Affects* (London: Routledge).

Batchelor, S. (1997) *Buddhism without Beliefs: A Contemporary Guide to Awakening* (London: Bloomsbury).

Batchelor, M. (2001) *Women on the Buddhist Path* (London: Thorsons).

Batchelor, M. (2007) *Let go: A Buddhist Guide to Breaking Free of Habits* (Somerville, MA: Wisdom).

Batchelor, S. (2010) *Confession of a Buddhist Atheist* (New York: Spiegel & Grau).

Bazzano, M. (2012) *Spectre of the Stranger: Towards a Phenomenology of Hospitality* (Eastbourne: Sussex Academic Press).

Brotto, L. and Barker, M. (2013) 'Special Issue on Mindful Sexual and Relationship Therapy', *Sexual & Relationship Therapy*, 28(1–2).

Brotto, L. A., Krychman, M. and Jacobson, P. (2008) 'Eastern Approaches for Enhancing Women's Sexuality: Mindfulness, Acupuncture, and Yoga', *Journal of Sexual Medicine*, 5, 2741–8.

Carrette, J. and King, R. (2005) *Selling Spirituality: The Silent Takeover of Religion* (London: Routledge).

Carson, J. W., Carson, K. M., Gil, K. M. and Baucom, D. H. (2004) 'Mindfulness Based Relationship Enhancement', *Behavioral Therapy*, 35, 471–94.

Chödrön, P. (1994) *The Places That Scare You: A Guide to Fearlessness* (London: HarperCollins).

Chödrön, P. (2001) *The Wisdom of no Escape: How to Love Yourself and Your World* (London: HarperCollins).

Cohen, E. (2010) 'From the Bhodi Tree, to the Analyst's Couch, Then Into the MRI Scanner: The Psychologisation of Buddhism', *Annual Review of Critical Psychology*, 8, 97–119.

Crane, R. (2009) *Mindfulness-based Cognitive Therapy* (London: Routledge).

Flaxman, P. E., Blackledge, J. T. and Bond, F. W. (2011) *Acceptance and Commitment Therapy* (London: Routledge).

Foucault, M. (1975) *Discipline and Punish*, translated by A. Sheridan (Harmondsworth: Penguin).

Fox, N. (2012) *The Body* (Cambridge: Polity Press).

Gergen, K. J. (2000) *The Saturated Self* (New York: Basic Books).

Gergen, K. (2009) *Relational Being: Beyond Self and Community* (Oxford: Oxford University Press).

Gilbert, P. (2010) *Compassion Focused Therapy* (London: Routledge).

Goldmeier, D. and Mears, A. J. (2010) 'Meditation: A Review of its use in Western Medicine and, in Particular, its Role in the Management of Sexual Dysfunction', *Current Psychiatry Review*, 6(1), 11–14.

Hanh, T. N. (1975) *The Miracle of Mindfulness* (Boston, MA: Beacon Press).

Hayes, S. (2005) *Get Out of Your Mind and Into Your Life: The New Acceptance and Commitment Therapy* (Oakland, CA: New Harbinger).

Kleinplatz, P. J. (2003) 'What's New in Sex Therapy: From Stagnation to Fragmentation', *Sex and Relationship Therapy*, 18, 95–106.

Kutchins, H. and Kirk, S. A. (1997) *Making us Crazy* (London: Constable).

Loy, D. (2008) *Money, Sex, War, Karma: Notes for a Buddhist Revolution* (Boston, MA: Wisdom Publications).

Magid, B. (2008) *Ending the Pursuit of Happiness* (Boston, MA: Wisdom Publications).

Pilgrim, D. (2010) 'The Diagnosis of Mental Health Problems', in Barker, M., Vossler, A. and Langdridge, D. (eds) *Understanding Counselling and Psychotherapy*, pp. 21–43 (London: SAGE).

Relate (2013) 'Relationship Counselling', available at: http://www.relate.org.uk/relationship-counselling/index.html (accessed 3 February 2013).

Richards, C. and Barker, M. (2013) *Sexuality and Gender for Counsellors, Psychologists and Health Professionals: A Practical Guide* (London: SAGE).

Segal, Z. V., Williams, J, M. G. and Teasdale, J. D. (2002) *Mindfulness-based Cognitive Therapy for Depression: A New Approach to Preventing Relapse* (New York: Guildford press).

Stanley, S. (2012) 'Mindfulness: Towards a Critical Relational Perspective', *Social and Personality Psychology Compass*, 6(9), 631–706.

Stanley, S., Barker, M. and Edwards, V. (in press) 'Swimming Against the Stream: Investigating Psychosocial Flows Through Mindful Awareness', *Qualitative Research in Psychology*.

Suttie, J. (2013) 'Can Mindfulness Treat Sexual Dysfunction', available at: http://greatergood.berkeley.edu/article/item/mindfulness_treat_sexual_dysfunction (accessed 1 February 2013).

Varela, F. J., Thompson, E. and Rosch, E. (1991) *The Embodied Mind: Cognitive Science and Human Experience* (London: MIT Press).

Walser, R. D. and Westrup, D. (2009) *The Mindful Couple* (Oakland, CA: New Harbinger Publications).

Wellwood, J. (1996) *Love and Awakening* (London: HarperCollins).

Williams, J. M. G. and Kabat-Zinn, J. (eds) (2011) 'Special Issue on Mindfulness', *Contemporary Buddhism*, 12(1), 1–306.

7
Mindfulness as a Secular Spirituality

Alex Gooch

Introduction

While a secular form of mindfulness may well be an effective problem-solving technique, it is incapable of addressing the more fundamental spiritual needs of the contemporary West; indeed, if it is taken as an ethic to live by, it is liable to make matters worse rather than better. Hence, this chapter will begin with some brief, general observations on the spiritual landscape of the West over the last hundred years, before considering mindfulness and its particular appeal in the contemporary Western world. In the final section, the limitations and potential dangers of mindfulness as a spiritual philosophy will be examined.

The Context of Post-modernity

The term 'mindfulness' clearly has its roots in Buddhist ideas and practices; it entered contemporary discourse as a translation of the term *sati*, a key term in the foundational Buddhist texts of the Pali Canon. However, both the word 'mindfulness' and the practice of cultivating it have been, at least to some extent, 'secularised out' of their Buddhist context—therapists and practitioners of many different hues today employ 'mindfulness' in a wide variety of ways, often without making any reference to Buddhist ideas at all. 'Secular' is derived from the Latin *saeculum*, meaning 'generation', 'lifetime', or 'historical period; hence, a 'secular spirituality' can be understood not only as a spirituality divorced from its traditionally 'religious' context, but also as a response to the particular spiritual needs and challenges of the times (Batchelor, 2012).

For my purposes here, the spiritual condition of the West in the early twenty-first century will be understood to be the condition known very broadly as 'post-modernity.' One of my contentions is that post-modernity constitutes an unresolved spiritual crisis; we are in the throes of this crisis right now, and at a cultural level we are grasping for possible solutions.

I define post-modernity, very crudely, as (in Lyotard's famous words) "incredulity towards grand narratives" (1984: xxiv). What, then, is a grand narrative? Scholars and academics have devoted decades to teasing out fine distinctions of meaning within this term; however, I intend to operate on another very crude definition of a 'grand narrative' as a set of beliefs, which together tell us about what the world *is*, what is true and false, what is good and bad, and so on. Clear examples of grand narratives might include medieval Christianity, or Soviet Communism, or contemporary Western secular liberalism.

Of course, grand narratives can overlap, and there are grand narratives within grand narratives, and so on; these issues need not detain us here. However, it is crucial to observe that a grand narrative is two things: it is an overarching and impersonal 'story' about how the world is put together, and it is also a framework within which I can tell my own story, as a discrete individual being with a past and a future. The grand narrative gives me an account of the particular causal relations that obtain between the 'ten thousand things' of the world; in other words, it tells me what is capable of causing what. Thus, it provides the matrix within which my own individual 'narrative identity'—my sense of my life as a story—is constituted. Furthermore, a satisfactory grand narrative must have an ethical aspect; that is, it must tell me what is right and wrong, good and bad, appropriate and inappropriate, and thus provide the ethical parameters and motivations around which I can structure the story of my life.

The grand narratives into which we are born constitute the existential ground under our feet; it is in terms of these grand narratives that our lives are comprehensible and meaningful. The doctrines, ideas, and assumptions that make up the grand narrative must be considered true—while other, competing or contradictory doctrines and ideas and assumptions must be considered false—if the grand narrative is to give shape and support to our lives. However, as we have observed, the defining characteristic of our own age is an attitude of 'incredulity' towards grand narratives.

Since time immemorial, the grand narratives that contained individual human lives were underwritten primarily by the authority of tradition. However, beginning in the Renaissance, the authority of tradition came to seem an inadequate basis for knowledge; scientists and other intellectual explorers began to seek to ground their ideas about the nature of the world (their grand narratives, in other words) not merely in received doctrine, but in the observations they could make with their own senses, and the inferences they could draw with their own reason.

To Doubt Everything

Seen through the eyes of critical reason, no belief is sacrosanct; all ideas can and must be subjected to critical investigation and potential deconstruction. This new attitude was given its systematic expression by René Descartes, who began his philosophical investigations with an explicit intention and willingness to doubt *everything*. Descartes' methodological assumption—that no statement is exempt from doubt and testing—signalled the end of our easy dwelling within our grand narratives. To dwell within a grand narrative, I must confidently believe that my grand narrative corresponds to the truth of how things *really* are. But if all ideas can and must be subjected to criticism and deconstruction, then the possibility of secure, confident belief in a meta-narrative is excluded right from the beginning, by the very nature of the enquiry. If *all* things are open to disproof, then even my most cherished belief is open to disproof—and even if my most cherished belief has stood for a thousand years, it may be disproved tomorrow. My human need to know the world and my place in it remains, but now my existential security is subject to the constant undermining anxiety that I may be wrong.

Since Descartes, the trajectory of Western thought has taken us further and further away from confident belief in our grand narratives, and deeper and deeper into the territory of uncertainty and doubt. In philosophy, Immanuel Kant tore down the assumption that there is a 'way things are, independently of us' (Stanford Encyclopedia of Philosophy, 2008), and Friedrich Nietzsche (1976), often invoked as the prophet of post-modernity, taught that there are, in fact, no 'facts' at all, only interpretations. The same movement away from certainty was visible in the advances made in physics in the twentieth century, which revealed a world that is not remotely conducive to confident, common-sense human understanding, and which (at least according to the Copenhagen interpretation) (Stanford Encylopedia of Philosophy, 2008) cannot properly be understood in terms of a single, unified, objective reality behind the appearances of things.

At the same time, developments in transport and communication lead to greater day-to-day awareness of and involvement with other cultures. Previously, we had been more able to go on with the view that our way of understanding the world was the only really serious way of understanding the world, and the grand narratives of distant communities and cultures were just colourful eccentricities in the margins, not really worth taking seriously. However, as communications technology developed, people were forced to contemplate the possibility that the world views of the Muslims, the Hindus, the Confucians, or even the Buddhists, might be just as sophisticated, and perhaps even just as valid, as their own.

Tolstoy declared that only one question is important for us: "What shall we do, and how shall we live?" (Weber, 1958: 143) At most times in human history, in most places in the world, this question would never have arisen; one would have lived and died securely in the embrace of a grand narrative, underpinned by the authority of ancestral tradition, which would have obviated the need to ever ask such a question. Of course, grand narratives do not keep anyone safe from moral dilemmas and conflict of conscience. However, Tolstoy's question speaks of more than just moral dilemmas; it expresses a vertiginous awareness that the foundations of ethical meaning are unreliable, and may already have given way. We might say that it is characteristic of post-moderns like us that we are able to ask Tolstoy's question—and that we are compelled to ask it, anxiously and urgently.

Secular Mindfulness

It may well be that we turn to a secular spiritual practice like mindfulness in the hope that it will tell us what we should do and how we should live—or at least that it will break the sense of existential deadlock that has come to accompany the question. I intend to consider the practice of secular mindfulness in terms of two key attitudes which it preaches: the focus on the present moment, and the 'de-centred' or 'de-centring' perspective (Crane, 2009; Alidina, 2010).

The first of these, the focus on the present moment, is relatively uncomplicated. The mindfulness practitioner is encouraged to keep bringing his or her attention back to the immediate experience of what is happening right now, rather than contemplating the past or the future, or engaging in daydreaming or abstract thought (Kabat-Zinn, 1990). 'De-centring' is rather more subtle; this term denotes an attitude of detachment from a particular thought or mental content. De-centring involves a re-drawing of the dividing line between subject and object; phenomena that are normally understood to be constitutive of the observing subject—thoughts, impulses, emotional states, and so on—are, from the 'de-centred' point of view, regarded not as features of the observing subject, but as objects to be observed.

For example, I normally understand my thoughts to be part of 'me'—but if I practice mindfulness, I am instructed to observe my thoughts, and in order to observe my thoughts I must place them outside myself, in the world 'out there', as objects of observation, rather than as the means for observing.

At this point, it is important to observe that mindfulness can be understood and presented in two distinct ways. First, there is what we might call 'problem-solving mindfulness'—mindfulness as a technique for addressing particular problematic mental contents or patterns. In distinction to this, there is the style of mindfulness practice that I shall call 'spiritual mindfulness', and which constitutes an existential or ethical orientation not only towards specific problematic mental contents, but towards the whole of life.

Both forms of mindfulness involve a deliberate re-drawing of the dividing line between subject and object, but they re-draw the line in crucially different places. The first form, 'problem-solving mindfulness', begins by identifying certain particular states of mind or psychological contents that are unwanted. It then reclassifies *only these* unwanted mental phenomena as external to the subject and as proper objects of detached observation. Other mental contents are not de-centred in the same way. Thus, for example, if I am a smoker trying to give up, I might 'mindfully' pay attention to my desire to smoke, observing in detail and in real time the particular thoughts, impulses, and so on that constitute this desire. I would observe that these thoughts and impulses are only passing phenomena; I would observe their rising and dying away, and thus, hopefully, their addictive hold over me would decrease over time. I would *not* mindfully observe my desire to give up smoking in the same way.

The goals of 'problem-solving mindfulness' are thus modest. This practice does not attempt to question the nature of the self per se; it attempts only to address and ameliorate specific unwanted states of mind. It is certainly not my intention here to call into question the effectiveness of mindfulness as a problem-solving technique; I am quite happy to concede that it is extremely effective in tackling a wide variety of problems.

However, mindfulness preached and practised in this way begs a deeper philosophical question. In order to practice this kind of selective mindfulness I must regard some of my internal contents as 'me' (e.g., the desire to give up smoking) and some as 'not-me' (e.g., the desire to smoke)—and mindfulness itself provides me with no principled grounds for making this distinction. In order to use mindfulness as a means for the solution of problems in my life, I must already have decided which elements of my mental experience constitute 'problems' and which elements do not. I must already have decided what I want to change about myself. In other words, in order to practice mindfulness-as-problem-solving-technique I must first have decided what I shall do and how I shall live.

If I come to mindfulness practice with a practical problem such as an addiction to nicotine, then all well and good, a 'problem-solving mindfulness' approach may very well help me to achieve my goal. But if I come with a more 'spiritual' problem—if I come with some variation of the overarching secular spiritual problem, an uncertainty regarding what I should do and how I should live—then 'problem-solving mindfulness' is not going to be equipped to help me.

What I am calling the 'spiritual mindfulness' approach is typically expressed in terms such as, for example, 'Practice is paying attention to thoughts without getting lost in them. Instead, we simply notice that thinking is taking place.' The above example is typical of *vipassana*-oriented meditation; a survey of self-help or popular spiritual literature would yield plenty more examples of the same idea expressed in similar terms. As the quotation illustrates, this form of mindfulness teaching does *not* say 'observe *some of* your thoughts, but only the ones you don't wish to entertain'—they say 'observe your thoughts', implying, 'observe *all* your thoughts, not only some of them.' If I come to mindfulness practice asking what I should do and how I should live, then I am likely to take the teachers at their word. And mindfulness can, indeed, be seen as offering answers to these questions. What shall I do? I shall dwell in the present moment, and take a de-centred stance towards my thoughts and internal experiences, not only some of them, but all of them. How shall I live? I shall live mindfully, to the very best of my ability, and I shall at least aim to be practising mindfulness every moment of every day.

This kind of 'general mindfulness', as an exclusive and thoroughgoing application of the principles of mindfulness, is much more profound and radical in its ambitions; it aims at a complete undercutting of the 'self' as normally understood and experienced.

So, if this latter form of mindfulness can be understood as a 'spirituality', we must next ask, how is 'secular'? How is it 'of the age'? The first answer is that it is secular in that it is Buddhism without a grand narrative. Buddhism in its traditional form, of course, *is* a grand narrative (or rather a family of more or less similar or related grand narratives), complete with metaphysics, ethics, and so on. The modern West finds grand narratives indigestible; hence, mindfulness without metaphysics makes for a form of Buddhism acceptable in the eyes of post-moderns.

However, the appeal of mindfulness to the contemporary post-modern mind goes deeper than that. One of the central difficulties that we post-moderns face is that we feel compelled to understand ourselves in terms of stories. We don't know how *not* to tell stories about ourselves, even though (as inheritors of Kant and Nietzsche) we have a nasty, creeping suspicion that these stories are, in fact, fictions or fabrications, groundless, because the meta-narratives on which they are based are also groundless. We live in stories, but we do so guiltily, dimly aware that we are being dishonest with ourselves. The 'mindfulness attitude' towards time—focusing on the present moment, experiencing past and future as constituted of thought-processes occurring in the present moment—provides relief from this anxiety about narratives by bringing the practitioner into an 'eternal present' in which the narrative self is deconstructed before it can even arise. The practitioner of mindfulness cleaves to the present moment, and in the present moment there are no stories, and hence no anxiety about the authenticity of stories.

In the same way, we can't help having a 'perspective', a 'take' on the world; we can't help employing categories like 'true' and 'false', 'right' and 'wrong.' We know that these categories are broken—or, rather, we know now that they always *were* broken, and our knowledge of their brokenness cannot, in good conscience, be repressed. And yet, we cannot think outside these categories. Hence, we go on as if post-modernity had never happened, as if we still believe that real knowledge of the world was a real possibility—but in our bones we don't believe it, and again there is anxiety and guilt.

The practice of 'de-centring'—regarding thoughts and all other elements of the 'inner life' as objects of attention and thus as exterior to the perceiving subject—can soothe our post-modern anxiety about truth because it opens up a space in which we can set aside judgements of true and false, right and wrong. In mindfulness practice, I have the experience of not *needing* to know what is true and what is not, that is, of not needing to worry about whether the content of any given thought is 'true' or 'false', 'valid' or 'invalid', to be anxiously clung to as the precious truth or to be anxiously pushed away as dangerous misapprehension. Thus, all the anxiety attendant on the need for such judgements is, at least ideally, suspended. I don't need to grasp at my story about the world, and clutch at it like a drowning man clutching at a life belt. In mindfulness practice I observe that this treasured, problematic story is constituted simply of thoughts—and of feelings attendant on the thoughts—and I can simply let these thoughts and feelings go, and return to observing the rise and fall of my breath.

The Trouble with Mindfulness

Thus, for the practitioner of mindfulness, the meditation cushion provides a haven from the existential anxieties occasioned by the *saeculum*. However, there is a danger that it can also exacerbate these anxieties. Insofar as mindfulness deliberately cultivates the perspective whereby the narrative self is seen to be nothing but an illusion thrown up by a succession of mental phenomena occurring in the present moment—much as the action on the cinema screen is an illusion thrown up by a succession of motionless frames occurring in the present moment—mindfulness practice amounts to a deliberate and systematic deconstruction of the narrative self. Present-moment practice, applied rigorously, undercuts not only negative future-oriented emotions such as anxiety or despair, but also positive future-oriented emotions; hope, for example, is always future-oriented, and thus a wholeheartedly present moment orientation requires the deconstruction of hope.

Insofar as it deliberately cultivates the capacity to let thoughts, feelings, motivations, and other 'inner phenomena' come and go, without identifying with them or acting upon them, mindfulness also amounts to a deconstruction of belief. It does not merely permit the abandonment of old, limiting beliefs, in order to make way for new, more expansive, or more wholesome beliefs; rather, by making the meditator conscious of the way that belief is constructed on a moment-by-moment basis, it attacks the very foundations of belief and makes it impossible.

These deconstructions may work very well on the cushion, but they do not necessarily remain on the cushion. Having once had direct meditative insight into the 'illusory' constitution of the self, or the arising-and-passing nature of ideas, one can never quite go back to one's earlier, naïve perceptions of the self as solid and substantial, and of one's ideas about the world as corresponding with the world itself. And it seems quite likely that the more one deconstructs one's narrative self and one's capacity for belief on the cushion in order to reside in mindfulness, the less solid one's narrative self and one's picture of the world will come to seem in the rest of life, when one is off the cushion and living an active life in the world.

Thus, mindfulness practice is in danger of contributing to our secular anxieties—and the more our secular anxieties increase, the more likely we are to take refuge from them on the meditation cushion. We must then ask what it would look like if someone really did take mindfulness, thus defined, as their primary guiding ethic and actually lived according to these principles 24/7.

One day in 1896, in a vault beneath the main temple at Tiruvannamalai in Tamil Nadu, southern India, a group of devotees came upon a young man sitting cross-legged in meditation. When he was discovered, he had apparently been sitting there for some time; he had been bitten by ants and rats, and pelted with stones by a gang of local children who had found him, but none of this seemed to interrupt his meditative practice. This young man would become famous as the Vedantic saint Sri Ramana Maharshi (Natarajan, 2006).

It is not clear exactly what kind of meditative exercise the saint-to-be was engaged in, but he might very well have been practising mindfulness. He might very well have been simply observing his thoughts, sensations, desires, motivations, and so on with calm detachment, allowing each one to arise and pass away without grasping at them or identifying with them or believing them, regarding them as no more constitutive of 'himself' than the birdsong or the wind in the trees.

Sitting in this state of perfect equanimity and dis-identification for hours and days at a stretch, Maharshi was gradually dying of hunger and thirst. Presumably, he was applying the principles of mindfulness consistently, and simply observing hunger and thirst when they arose, allowing them to be present if they were present, not passing judgement on them, but also not identifying with them or believing them, not allowing them to drag him out of the present moment into future-oriented concerns about his health and bodily well-being.

In fact, his discoverers poured water and food into his mouth and managed to get him to swallow it, and eventually brought him back to at least a certain degree of engagement with the world. However, left to his own devices, it seems that he might well have sat there in the lotus posture on the floor of the temple cellar until he keeled over and, with perfect equanimity, died.

I contend that death on the cushion would be entirely consistent with the principles of 'spiritual mindfulness'; indeed, if applied with absolute rigour, the logic of 'spiritual mindfulness' must lead, inevitably, to disengagement, absolute passivity, literal motionlessness, and eventual death from neglect of the body's needs. I do not find this an inspiring ideal, and I venture to assume that the reader does not either.

Of course, Maharshi was a meditator of extraordinarily prodigious natural gifts. Lacking extreme capacity to regard our experience 'mindfully', most of us would surely be incapable of reaching the point he reached. Most of us would have buckled, got up from the cushion and gone to the fridge long before hunger or thirst reached physically dangerous levels. For the 'perfect practitioner', living according to the principles of mindfulness alone and able to apply them flawlessly in every moment, perfect inactivity and an unperturbed death on the cushion might be a possibility. For the 'imperfect practitioner' like you or me, the attempt to take mindfulness as an ethic to live by is liable not to overcome, but to exacerbate the spiritual problems of post-modernity that brought us to it in the first place. It is likely to pitch us deeper into the very disorientation and depression from which mindfulness as a circumscribed meditative practice provides temporary release.

I certainly do not intend to claim that mindfulness is bad, and should not be practised—only that mindfulness is not an adequate response to the secular question of "What shall we do and how shall we live?" Mindfulness will not obviate our need to have a reliably grounded sense of identity and nor will it provide solid ground on which to base our identities. It will not relieve us of our yearning to feel that we know what the world is in order to interact meaningfully with it—and nor will it restore our crumbling capacity to know what the world is.

'Present moment practice' and de-centring are both valuable, but in order to function as human beings in society we also require the precise opposites of these virtues; we require meaningful orientation towards the future, and we require beliefs (at least provisional ones) in order to orient ourselves towards the world and interact with it in a meaningful way. It is belief and the narrative self that have been rendered problematic by post-modernity, and while mindfulness may provide us with a 'night's shelter', it is not a convincing answer to our contemporary spiritual problems.

References

Alidina, S. (2010) *Mindfulness for Dummies* (Chichester: John Wiley & Sons).

Batchelor, S. (2012) 'A Secular Buddhist', available at: http://gaiahouse.co.uk/wp-content/uploads/Stephen-Batchelor-A-Secular-Buddhist.pdf (accessed 29 May 1 2013).

Crane, R. (2009) *Mindfulness-based Cognitive Therapy* (London: Routledge).

Kabat-Zinn, J. (1990) *Full Catastrophe Living. How to Cope With Stress, Pain and Illness Using Mindfulness Meditation* (London: Piatkus Books).

Lyotard, J. F. (1984) *The Postmodern Condition: A Report on Knowledge* (Minneapolis, MN: University of Minnesota).

Natarajan, A.R. (2006) *Timeless in Time: Sri Ramana Maharshi* (Bloomington, IN: World Wisdom).

Nietzsche, F. (1976) *The Portable Nietzsche* (W. Kaufmann trans., ed.) (Harmondsworth: Penguin).

Stanford Encyclopedia of Philosophy (2008) Copenhagen interpretation of quantum mechanics, available at: http://plato.stanford.edu/entries/qm-copenhagen (accessed 31 October 2013).

Weber, M. (1958) 'Science as a Vocation', in Gerth, H. H. and Wright Mills, C. (eds) *From Max Weber: Essays in Sociology* (New York: Oxford University Press).

8
Mindfulness and Therapy: A Skeptical Approach

Rebecca Greenslade

Introduction

Mindfulness-based approaches are the current mental health zeitgeist, shaped into therapeutic application through alignments with 'third wave' approaches such as mindfulness-based cognitive therapy (MBCT). The fact that they are, at present, accepted more or less univocally raises several questions, one of which pertains to the potential elevation of these approaches to the realm of the undisputed. Opening a discussion on the origins of *skepticism* in meditation practice and the field of therapy, I will suggest that the complementary relationship between the ancient philosophies of Pyrrhonian skepticism (Empiricus, 1990) and the Buddhist Madhyamaka school (Nāgārjuna, 1995) might provide a practical challenge to what may easily turn, if passively accepted, into a form of dogmatism. I will argue that the above offer the parameters for the construction of a therapeutic alliance that shifts us from a behavioral understanding of the self towards one encouraging a greater embodiment of the lived experience of both therapist and client. Both philosophies encourage a way of life that embodies the suspension of one's judgment and beliefs. This attitude potentially leads to freedom from mental conflict, or anxiety—an attitude that, as I will suggest, can be lacking in contemporary therapeutic applications of mindfulness-based approaches.

Towards a Skeptical Approach to Psychotherapy

A skeptical approach to psychotherapy (Heaton, 1993, 1999) adheres to a discourse of constructive challenge of theory and world view. As such, it emphasizes expediency over doctrine. Its roots lie in Pyrrhonian skepticism, which takes its name from the Greek philosopher Pyrrho of Elis (360–270 BC). Pyrrho did not write anything and we rely chiefly upon two main sources to provide us with an insight into his philosophy and life, informed, first, by the sketchy remnants of the writings of Timon of Philius, a contemporary of Pyrrho. Diogenes Laertius (2011) provides a biographical account of Pyrrho and insights into his philosophical attitude. Second, Sextus Empiricus, a philosopher, physician, and adherent of Pyrrhonian philosophical practices, writing in the latter part of the third century AD, provides a thorough presentation on the philosophy that informed his own skeptical attitude in *Outlines of Pyrrhonism* (1990).

Pyrrhonian philosophers were unique in the West in their attempts to differentiate the *non-evident* from the *evident* in human experience. They refused to develop beliefs about non-evident matters, for or against. For the Pyrrhonists, beliefs about things non-evident were inherently dogmatic as they could not be authenticated and therefore be accepted with any certainty. It was the ramifications of this lack of certainty, such as fear and anxiety, which was, according to the Pyrrhonists, the main source of human suffering (Kuzminski 2008). What Pyrrhonists questioned was not *what* appeared, but the judgments and beliefs we *hold* about appearances. We cannot claim to know *how* or *why* they appear. Consequently, rather than deny all claims, which would have been dogmatic, the Pyrrhonists advocated suspending judgment (*epoché*) about them. Once such judgments were suspended, they experienced a subsequent liberation from anxiety, at least relating to the uncertainty associated with the beliefs in question (ibid).

Pyrrhonian skeptics saw their philosophy as primarily therapeutic. Kuzminski describes Pyrrhonism, in its most basic terms, as "a therapeutic and liberating practice advocating no views" (2008: 2). It is a lifestyle (*agoge*) that leads to *ataraxia*, freedom from mental discord, or tranquility. As appearances are no longer limited by the beliefs typically held about them, they can now be valued for what they are—immediate, direct experiences unattached to suppositions or hypotheses. Annas and Barnes describe the skeptical position as one of "practical doubt" (1985: 9). Suspending judgment has an ameliorative outcome. However, Pyrrhonian skeptics emphasized that approaching *ataraxia* (tranquility) as something to be achieved or attained is a source of conflict in itself. It is not something to be strived for, but occurs inadvertently through the method of suspension of judgment. Sextus Empiricus used the following illustration:

> The skeptic, in fact, had the same experience which is said to have befallen the painter Apelles. Once, they say, when he was painting a

horse and wished to represent in the painting the horse's foam, he was so unsuccessful that he gave up the attempt and flung at the picture the sponge on which he used to wipe the paints off his brush, and the mark of the sponge produced the effect of a horse's foam (1990: 24–5).

Quietude emerged when Apelles relinquished the attempt of trying to paint the perfect representation of the horse's foam. *Epoché* cannot therefore be purposely attained, but occurs from an attitude of suspension of judgment. There appears to be a distinct contrast between the skeptical attitude of *epoché* and Husserl's later reductive, transcendental application, often referred to as 'bracketing' in psychotherapy practice. Husserl's understanding of *epoché* seems to be problematic in that it is caught up in *methodology* in contrast to the skeptical *method*. As Heaton (2003) points out, Husserl's *epoché* requires an act of will from the outset. Husserl instructs us to bracket our beliefs borne from the natural attitude in order to shift into the phenomenological attitude, where the ability to suspend judgment upon these beliefs occurs. It could be argued that his version of phenomenology is not entirely immune from dogmatism. Husserl replaces the set of beliefs inherent in the natural attitude with the belief that suspension of judgment can occur within the phenomenological attitude. In contrast, the Pyrrhonist has no epistemological construction within which to perform *epoché*. It is an example of the difference between embodying a philosophical attitude and applying a philosophical technique with a specific outcome in mind.

Pyrrho was known for his use of caveats and curious forms of speech, which had performative rather than indicative functions (Kuzminski, 2007). Through the use of counter-argumentation, Pyrrhonists would vanquish their opponents and then refute the argument they had used to destabilize their opponent's position. Diogenes Laertius details some of the well-known Pyrrhonian admonitions, including "every reason has a corresponding reason opposed to it" and "not more one thing or another" and "prudence has not existence, any more than it has no existence" (2011: 255). What is distinct about the Pyrrhonian caveat is that it is not conclusive, but neutralizing. It does not close down the possibility of further argument, but leaves it open, suspending judgment upon the matters that are beyond direct experience, in contrast to reaching a definitive position (Kuzminski, 2007). As Sextus Empiricus writes,

> The main basic principle of the skeptic system is that of opposing to every proposition an equal proposition; for we believe that as a consequence of this we end by ceasing to dogmatize (1990: 19).

Sextus Empiricus uses the term 'skeptic' in its original sense from the Greek *skeptikos*, meaning 'inquiring' and 'reflective', although it later adopted a more general usage of someone who doubted the possibility of knowledge of any kind. Annas and Barnes (1985) make a distinction between the *practical skepticism* of Pyrrho and the *professional skepticism* of Arcesilaus of Pitane, who headed Plato's Academy and converted the school to (academic) skepticism. For the former, counter-arguing was a way of life; for the latter, skepticism became part of a professional philosophy concerned with epistemological issues and fundamental philosophical questions. Sextus Empiricus (1990) emphasizes that whilst Pyrrhonism is a philosophical position, it is inherently practical, moving beyond academic exercise into a way of life. It is, perhaps, this emphasis that makes the goal of *ataraxia* unique to Pyrrhonian skepticism. Whilst similarities have been drawn between *ataraxia* and Democritus' notion of *euthumia*, literally meaning cheerfulness, it seems unlikely that Democritus' usage carries the liberating connotations associated with suspension of judgment (Flintoff, 1980). Pyrrhonists appear to have placed greater emphasis upon suspension of judgment as a prerequisite for gaining *ataraxia*, to the extent that they suspended judgment on their own suspension of judgment.

Implications for Psychotherapy

What, however, are the implications of a skeptical attitude for a psychotherapist? It seems to me that there is much to be gained for both therapist and client. Clients bring their beliefs to psychotherapy. Beliefs provide us with security amidst uncertainty; they shape our values, choices, experiences, and self-perceptions. The function of beliefs is latent within the therapeutic industry itself. Since Freud's tripartite model of the human psyche (1991), different therapeutic approaches have been competing in epistemologic and scientific methodologies. It could be argued that each approach is concerned with the dogmatism of 'truth', of finding models we believe we can match our clients to and design appropriate treatment plans to relieve them of their symptoms. Broadly speaking, Freud's system of belief was the assumption of the unconscious as the source of repression and behavioral anomalies. To reveal the 'truth', we must unravel and re-program our unconscious mechanisms. Yet, the 'truth' depends upon the therapeutic model the client is subjected to, and influences the terms and conditions upon how the client understands their experiences (Heaton, 2003). A skeptical psychotherapist will endeavor to suspend judgment upon their own theoretical orientation, listening with openness and wonder to their clients. As Heaton describes:

> The skeptics argued...that to be convinced of a truth does not make it a truth...So the skeptical therapist refrains from giving his assent to the truth or falsehood of these imaginary constructions, he wants to help the patient see beyond meaning and sense (2003: 38).

Through refusing to respond to clients' beliefs as 'truths', the skeptical psychotherapist invites the client to free themselves from the identifications they might hold of themselves and others. They will encourage their clients to question beliefs and to develop their own antimonies and caveats through which self-understanding may be furthered. Through relinquishing attachments to beliefs, clients may well experience the lessening of difficult and painful emotions associated with such beliefs, such as fear and anxiety. The following statement from Kuzminski on the Pyrrhonian attitude towards beliefs seems pertinent to the therapeutic endeavor:

> Beliefs, after all, project the believer into a hypothetical future whose emotional resonance can become the dominant experience of the present, giving rise to undue excitement and anxiety. We see this in obsession and other forms of psychic pathology. Absent such beliefs, the emotional resonance dissolves and tranquillity is able to supervene, or so the Pyrrhonists claimed (2008: 13).

Pyrrhonism and Buddhism

Pyrrho accompanied Alexander the Great's voyage to the East and it was this journey and likely meetings with Indian 'holy men' that influenced his skeptical philosophy. Flintoff's (1980) formative paper 'Pyrrho in India' sets out the argument for Buddhist influence in Pyrrhonian philosophy. It is an argument that has been extended by Kuzminski's more recent work (2007, 2008). Flintoff (1980) describes the main similarity between Pyrrhonian and Buddhist thought to be the antithetical attitude towards all things metaphysical and all assertions. Polarity and antimony is found in the earliest Buddhist sutras, and the Buddha was known for using these to assume an agnostic position towards all metaphysical questions. Flintoff writes:

Had he [the Buddha]...given a 'yes' or 'no' answer, he would have been guilty of the very dogmatism (*ditthi*) which he so consistently condemned in others...Criticism is deliverance of the human mind from all entanglements and passions. It is freedom itself (1980: 92).

Criticism, or reflective capacity, lies at the heart of Buddhist teaching. This is evidenced through the teachings of Nāgārjuna (1995), in particular, who is credited with originating the Madhyamaka school. This is strikingly similar to Pyrrho's position that suspension of judgment upon all things non-evident leads to an unperturbed experience of mind and is a vehicle towards liberation. Kuzminski (2007) goes further, suggesting that *epoché* can be recognized in the Madhyamaka teaching of emptiness. Through suspending judgment on non-evident assertions, we are left only with what is evident, now empty of any judgmental content. As Nāgārjuna says, "emptiness is the relinquishing of all views. For whomever emptiness is a view, that one will accomplish nothing" (XIII.8: 36, quoted in Kuzminski, 2007: 498). Suspension of judgment, therefore, is an essential prerequisite to Buddhist liberation, or freedom from anxiety.

A second similarity between Pyrrhonian and Madhyamaka thought is the mode of argument called the *quadrilemma*. It translates roughly as, "We must not say about any one thing (1) that it is or (2) that it is not or (3) that it is and is not or (4) that it is neither or not" (Flintoff, 1980: 92). The quadrilemma is a philosophical configuration of possibilities: a positive hypothesis and a negative counter-hypothesis, which are combined to create a third alternative and separated to create a fourth. An example of its use in Buddhism can be found in Nāgārjuna's teachings: "Everything is real and is not real, both real and not real, neither real nor not real. This is the Lord Buddha's teaching" (XVIII. 8: 49, quoted in Kuzminski, 2008: 56). It was used widely by various Indian schools, including Buddhists and Jains, and, possibly, the early Indian skeptic Sankara. However, Flintoff's assertion that the quadrilemma was unique to Indian philosophy may be questionable. Kuzminski (2007) refers to Hankinson's reminder that Aristotle mentions the quadrilemma in his *Metaphysics* (expressing his frustration at those who used it). Yet what is perhaps unique about the Pyrrhonian and Indian schools of thought's use of this method is that it was for the purpose of liberation rather than academic dispute. The intention of these antinomies, in both Buddhist and Pyrrhonian thinking, is that through their articulation, tranquility ensues. Flintoff makes the important point that the attainment of 'enlightenment' in Buddhism is by no means as direct as it is in Pyrrhonism. There are a number of central ideas, such as the Four Noble Truths and the Eight Fold Path, which hold no Pyrrhonian equivalent. However, both philosophies use antinomian argument to transform their experience of the world into one of tranquility:

> A cessation of all conceptualization (*epoché*) takes place which leads onto a cessation of speech (*aphasia*) which lead in turn to a cessation of all troubledness (*ataraxia, nirvana, moksa*) (1980: 94).

Through an understanding of the function of antimonies, we can see that both Pyrrhonism and the Madhyamaka hold a comparable attitude towards beliefs and appearances. Both appear to accept the immediate evidence of the senses and thought as they appear to us. For Pyrrhonists, a belief is a dogmatic assertion that something exists beyond what appears to us. Similarly, Madhyamaka philosophy does not teach that anything exists in this sense. For Kuzminski,

> The Madhyamaka, like Pyrrhonism, is distinguished precisely by its radical skepticism, by its refusal to countenance any sort of statement or belief, positive or negative, even to the point of calling into question the fundamental tenets of traditional Buddhism itself. What the Pyrrhonists call 'dogmatism' ('dogma,' from *dokeo*, that which seems to be true), Buddhists, it would appear, call 'attachment,' or 'clinging' (*upādāna*) to a fixed 'view' (*drsti*); this means the positing of hidden, unclear, but unconditional and determining entities, so-called 'true' realities, which are said to govern our experience (2007: 498).

Equally striking to the doctrinal similarities are the practical ones, and the extent to which both Pyrrhonism and Buddhism are philosophies *to be lived*. An illustration is Pyrrho's acceptance of and ability to endure pain (Laertius, 2011). Whilst the ability to self-anesthetize was unheard of in Greece, it was common practice for the Indian yogi, who, through the practice of various yoga postures (*asanas*), cultivated greater control over the suffering of the body and mind (Flintoff, 1980: 98). Diogenes tells a number of stories that illustrate the extent to which Pyrrho embodied indifference and non-involvement, for example walking past his mentor, Anaxarchus, when he had fallen into a pond without helping him, carrying poultry, washing pigs, and cleaning furniture—acts which, typically, a man of his status would not have carried out. Diogenes also describes Pyrrho adopting an itinerant, ascetic lifestyle upon his return to Greece, similar to the wandering

Indian *sannyasins* whose lack of attachment to the world is represented through the renunciation of their homes and the severing of family ties. Whilst some Greek philosophers were known to roam in the neighboring mountains, such as Heraclitus and Socrates, Flintoff (1980) suggests that they nonetheless retained their political involvement with their native cities, whereas Pyrrho's ascetic lifestyle was distinguished by his political disengagement.

Pyrrhonian skepticism requires an *ability* to dialectically challenge non-evident belief. What is not immediately evident in Pyrrho's practical application of his philosophy is meditation. It is unlikely he would not have been exposed to various contemplative practices during his time in India, yet his philosophy advocated verbal antimonies rather than non-verbal practices. In meditation, one observes the immediate experiences that arise and pass, such as thoughts or emotions, neither trying to alter them or become involved in them. It is through non-involvement that we can see beliefs for what they are and free ourselves from their hold. It might be reasonable, therefore, to see Pyrrho's practical philosophy as congenial with meditation practice.

In Ancient Greece spiritual exercises (*askesis*) were an important part of progressing in philosophical wisdom. Theory was not seen as an end in itself but put in the service of practice (Hadot, 1995). It seems likely, therefore, that Pyrrho's emphasis on philosophy as a way of life did not belong solely to Indian influences. The emphasis on meditation as a practice to abandon attachment to beliefs is, of course, unambiguous in Nāgārjuna's philosophy, where we find statements such as "By abandoning, that is not abandoned. Abandonment happens through meditation" (1995: XVII. 15: 45) and "The cessation of ignorance occurs through meditation" (1995: XXVI 11: 78).

There are significant similarities between Pyrrhonism and the Madhyamaka. What might a comparison of two ancient practical philosophical systems mean for a practitioner contemplating the use of contemporary mindfulness approaches within therapeutic contexts?

Towards a Mindfulness-based Skeptical Psychotherapy

Mindfulness-based approaches emerged in the UK through the introduction of MBCT in the 1990s. It combines aspects of cognitive behavioral therapy (CBT) with the straightforward practice of mindfulness—bringing our awareness to the present moment, purposefully and without judgment. Mindfulness is a way of being—a capacity for moment-by-moment awareness. There are numerous research studies that suggest the positive effect a regular meditation practice can have on one's health and well-being. Certainly, as I began my own meditation practice a few years ago, I have experienced greater ease and joy in my life. I consider my practice to be inseparable from my work with clients in how it supports me be present with them and their difficulties.

Yet, accompanying this enthusiasm for the therapeutic benefits of mindfulness is a concern that its application is becoming removed from the philosophical and practical contexts from which it emerged (Bazzano, 2010). Through neglecting the many possible connections between ancient contemplative practices and their contemporary therapeutic application, are we possibly limiting what we offer to clients? Separating mindfulness from its Buddhist context can be helpful in broadening its appeal and accessibility across health care professions. Yet, mindfulness it is often presented as a technique that can solve our problems.

I would suggest that life's predicaments are not to be solved: they are inherent to the human condition. Through the practice of meditation, we cultivate a positively skeptical attitude that recognizes with greater clarity the situation we find ourselves in at any given time. The therapeutic quality of mindfulness lies in seeing experiences as they appear and suspending judgment on the beliefs we attach to them. Batchelor (2011) emphasizes that meditation cannot be reduced to a proficiency in technique, but that it is the cultivation of a *sensibility*—our response to being-in-the-world.

Personal experiences that echoed these concerns motivated me to write this chapter. During an eight-week MBCT course a few years ago, I was struck by the distinctly 'un-skeptical' spirit of the course and its emphasis on what Bazzano describes as its 'normative' elements, that is, a focus on using meditation to reframe 'negative' thoughts and behaviors (2010: 36). There was an emphasis on imparting knowledge and techniques, rather than on experiencing. At times, it felt as if the facilitators' loyalty to their weekly teaching agenda restricted them somewhat and made them less open and, on the whole, uninterested in suspending judgment and staying with the questions participants raised, hastening instead to soothe issues emerging from the class. I left with a feeling of overall dissatisfaction. I couldn't help feeling that the quality of self-discovery of an embodied meditation practice had been replaced with an emphasis on self-improvement and adjustment.

Last year, I attended a week-long teacher's training retreat to learn how to facilitate mindfulness and meditation groups. I was struck by the number of participants on the course who did not have a regular meditation practice. Many were unfamiliar with meditation. They were attending with the understanding that they would learn how to teach meditation techniques. Whilst a committed and regular meditation practice was emphasized, it was not a pre-requisite. In a similar vein, a friend of mine—an experienced clinical psychologist—recently contacted me as she had been asked to start including mindfulness in her work with serious violent offenders and wanted to know if I could provide any good exercises that she could 'do' with her clients.

These instances are a far cry from the cultivation of a *sensibility* that Batchelor (2011) emphasizes. Its therapeutic benefits were originally conceived and imparted through the embodied practices of the Buddha and his enquiry into the existential human condition. One cannot but question how a client can cultivate mindfulness as a way of life if this practice is not, to at least some degree, embodied in those they learn from.

In reading the first edition of *Mindfulness-Based Cognitive Therapy for Depression* by Segal et al. (2002), I was struck by their account of how—despite being established practitioners and researchers in CBT—their own assumptions and beliefs were profoundly challenged and revised when considering the relationship of CBT to mindfulness and its therapeutic application. These shifts in understanding emerged from their own observations of the facilitation of the well-established mindfulness-based stress reduction (MBSR) program in Massachusetts, USA.

Through observing MBSR facilitators, they came to identify the crucial importance of the facilitators' own practice of mindfulness, something they had dismissed in their original conception. The effect of this was twofold. First, through their own experience, facilitators were able to relate to the experiences of their clients. Interestingly, the roles of client (seeking help) and facilitator (offering help) were abandoned. Second, instead of trying to provide solutions to issues raised by clients, MBSR facilitators were instead *inviting* clients to bring these problems into their awareness and simply breathe into them. This shifted the focus from fixing to experiencing. As Segal et al. write,

> We had now seen for ourselves the remarkable way they were able to embody a different relationship to the most intense distress and emotion in their patients. And we had seen the MBSR instructors going further in their work with negative affect than we had been able to...by staying in our therapist roles. We now saw more clearly how these two things were connected: that this ability to relate differently to negative affect came from having their own ongoing mindfulness practice, so that they might teach mindfulness out of their experience

of it. A vital part of what the MBSR instructor conveyed was his or her own embodiment of mindfulness in interactions with the class (2002: 56).

An equally significant shift was in their understanding of how we relate to thoughts and feelings. Traditionally, CBT makes a causal connection between negative thinking and depression. The therapist will invite the client to record negative thoughts as they occur, to be evaluated and rigorously examined for their evidence. Over time, clients are taught skills and techniques that enable them to identify and challenge negative thoughts before a depression is triggered. However, rather than learning a set of skills, the development of MBCT was rooted in the invitation that clients simply recognize their thoughts as thoughts and feelings as feelings. Instead of getting involved in the beliefs they held about them, they were invited to simply observe their relationship towards them, as the experience occurred. In many ways, MBCT is about cultivating an embodied attitude towards experience, rather than trying to change it and, in this respect, it seems to have sincere alignments to a skeptical form of psychotherapy. Although MBCT was born out of openness, embodiment, and an attitude of non-dogmatism, it still remains susceptible to these attitudes being lost through an excessive emphasis on technique.

Conclusion

A skeptical attitude invites us to engage in the spirit of enquiry, into an examination of phenomena devoid of attachment and over-involvement. It encourages clients to engage with their own experiences as they arise. We can cultivate this attitude through the practical application of particular philosophical positions, namely Pyrrhonism and Madhyamaka, and through their practical application philosophy can become a way of life. It can inform our therapeutic discourse with clients. Verbal caveats and counter-arguments encourage therapist and client to neutralize their beliefs and see things as they emerge. As an embodied practice of equanimity, meditation supports and develops suspension of judgment, allowing new possibilities to emerge. In terms of mindfulness-based approaches, a shift from the reductionism of mindfulness as a technique to mindfulness as a skeptical sensibility invites therapists and clients alike to explore a therapeutic way of life that cultivates tranquility over anxiety. As a psychotherapist, I find this both professionally and personally liberating.

References

Annas, J. and Barnes, J. (1985) *The Modes of Scepticism: Ancient Texts and Modern Interpretations* (Cambridge: Cambridge University Press).

Batchelor, S. (2011) 'The Phenomenology of Meditation, Part 1', lecture at Gaia House Zen retreat, available at: http://www.dharmaseed.org/teacher/169/talk/16036/ (accessed 4 November 2013).

Bazzano, M. (2010) 'Mindfulness in Context', *Therapy Today*, 21, 3, 33–6.

Empiricus, S. (1990) *Outlines of Pyrrhonism* (New York: Prometheus Books).

Flintoff, E. (1980) 'Pyrrho and India', *Phronesis* XXV, 2, 88–105.

Freud, S. (1991) *On Metapsychology* (London: Penguin).

Hadot, P. (1995) *Philosophy as Way of Life* (Oxford: Blackwell Publishing).

Heaton, J.M. (1993) 'The Sceptical Tradition in Psychotherapy', in Spurling, L. (ed.) *From the Words of my Mouth: Tradition in Psychotherapy*, pp. 106–31 (London: Routledge).

Heaton, J.M. (1999) 'Scepticism and Psychotherapy: A Wittgensteinian Approach', in Mace, C. (ed.) *Heart and Soul: The Therapeutic Face of Philosophy*, pp. 47–64 (London: Routledge).

Heaton, J.M. (2003) 'Pyrrhonian Scepticism and Psychotherapy', *Existential Analysis*, 14, 1, 32–47.

Kuzminski, A. (2007) 'Pyrrhonism and the Madhyamaka', *Philosophy East & West*, 57, 4, 482–511.

Kuzminski, A. (2008) *Pyrrhonism: How the Ancient Greeks Reinvented Buddhism* (Lanham, MD: Lexington Books).

Laertius, D. (2011) *The Lives and Opinions of Eminent Philosophers: Volume 2.* (Memphis, TN: General Books LLC).

Nāgārjuna (1995) (translation and commentary by. J. L. Garfield) *The Fundamental Wisdom of the Middle Way [Nāgārjuna's Mulamadhyamakakarika]* (Oxford: Oxford University Press).

Segal, Z. V., Williams, J, M. G. and Teasdale, J. D. (2002) *Mindfulness-based Cognitive Therapy for Depression: A New Approach to Preventing Relapse* (New York: Guildford Press).

9
Meditation and Meaning

Jeff Harrison

Introduction

If I were to write this chapter tomorrow, I would be different, the world would be different, and the chapter would be different. All is flux. Paradoxically, conventional theoretical statements—if they are to retain any enduring value—can only denote the unchanging qualities of such flux, perhaps by describing a mode of perception or quality of being, rather than its contents.

Meaning involves language: What can we say *about* meditation that does not run counter to the claims we might make for it? If meditation is defined as awareness of phenomenal arising, can theory—even theory that is light on its feet—ever translate such unpredictable and infinitely nuanced understanding into discourse?

There is no view from nowhere. It is equally true that there is no view from everywhere. When it comes to viewpoints, all is partial. In that sense, too, all theories and models of reality are reductive. The basics of our language can all too easily lull us into the sense that the world really is like that. This is the 'god of grammar.' Even the word 'process', often invoked to draw us away from instrumentalism, is a thing (i.e., a noun).

Language can be parsed; and it parses the world—it breaks it up into units. Wittgenstein (1972) noted our bewitchment by language. Rorty (1989) pointed up the rhetorical dimension of philosophy. But what can we do? Human beings *are* reflective; and there is no such thing as a meta-language that is not also a language. A liminological approach to words, one that is aware of pushing at the provisional and often misleading edges of meanings, is one possible solution (Wang, 2001).

So we have flux, partiality, and a degree of misdirection.

Attention, then, must be the watchword, as it is in meditation.

Unfolding and Enfoldedness

Merleau-Ponty, phenomenologist of embodied consciousness, wrote: "No philosophy can be ignorant of finitude, under pain of failing to understand itself as philosophy" (1962: 38). As we approach one horizon, another unfolds. The world is "an open and indefinite multiplicity of relationships, which are of reciprocal implication." (ibid: 71) Meditation can help us realise this situation of unfolding and enfoldedness. Language struggles to convey it. As we become empty of illusory—because separate—self, we open to the other.

A discourse of this kind cuts into the world to piece it back together again. "Any act of knowing", writes Flemons (1991: 1), "any knowing act, begins with the drawing of a distinction, with the noting of a difference... Knowing is composed of boundaries imposed." We might also recall Nietzsche's pertinent observation: "A critique of knowledge is senseless: how should a tool be able to criticise itself when it can use only itself for the critique?" (Lawson, 1985: 40). Merleau-Ponty chose what he called 'radical reflection' on, rather than analysis of, experience because the latter would require a form of synthesis to repair the damage it had itself done (Honderich, 1995).

Furthermore, language is also differential. It works by distinction. The common coin is two-sided. 'Self' means nothing without 'other'; so, if *all* is self (or other), then nothing is self (or other). Not only that: distinctions can be misleading in other ways. We might differentiate between nature and culture, yet we need to acknowledge that nature, when culturally perceived, is at least as much cultural as natural. There are distinctions, but there are also overlaps and takeovers.

Lenses and perspectives do matter then; they are at least as fundamental as what they purport to look at and describe. And yet the only way we can address them is via lenses and perspectives. We can be subtle, we can be liminological; but medium, viewpoint, and reference are intimately and intricately linked. We are, indeed, folded in. There is no neutral ground. We *know* this—and that is one of the reasons it is so readily overlooked.

If, as Bateson (2000) argues, it takes two to know one (given that solitary introspection is as unreliable game) then a 'double lens', or relationship of two tempts us to introduce a further vantage point because, as Keeney notes, "to know two, extending this logic of relationship, necessarily requires the presence of *three*" (Flemons, 1991: xi). Perhaps we just have to accept our limitations, at least in the face of what we can see and of what language can reliably designate. For even as we suggest alternatives to language, it is unlikely that those alternatives will be entirely impervious to it and, even if they are, we use language as the medium of our suggestion. Such observations can be unsettling, for our Western culture has a bias towards a singular, self-present, unitary, and disembodied consciousness predicated on Platonic and neo-Platonic thought, which fed into early Christianity.

Conversely, given its roots in the dharma, mindfulness ultimately sees the 'self' as de-centred, as fundamentally embodied and embedded in the world, seeking to get "one up on it" (Watts, 1975: 66). In that respect, the term 'mindfulness' is misleading, for it does not extrapolate a substantial and separate self (mind) from ever-changing, emergent phenomena, nor does it sustain self-defensive epistemologies as forms of mastery over the world/self. In the preface to *Phenomenology of Perception*, Merleau-Ponty (1962) suggests that we ascribe essences to the world to help us prevail over it. In mindfulness, mystery survives mastery.

Perhaps the most famous definition in the West of mindfulness is Kabat-Zinn's: "Mindfulness means paying attention in a particular way: on purpose, in the present moment, and non-judgmentally" (1994: 4). No one could, of course, predict or enumerate the contents of that awareness. There is a shift toward the perceptual and away from the conceptual. One begins to observe without proliferative commentary. There is a curious mixture of knowing and not-knowing in mindfulness: one is aware of the *minutiae* of phenomenal arising, but one does not seek to extrapolate from it into static model, framework or foundational theory. Self is envisaged as a *verb*, a process, *rather than a noun*. It is not only Western commentators whose descriptive language strains at the limits: for Thich Nhat Hanh, "mindfulness of feeling in feeling is the mind experiencing mindfulness of the mind in the mind" (1975: 41). Mindfulness is radical awareness and enquiry, fostering insight into phenomena, including—and especially—the illusion of stable, substantial selfhood.

So, where are we? We might ask this question in mindfulness practice, just as we might, for very different reasons, in a piece of discourse like this where 'we tend to envisage ourselves as surveying the material and marshalling the argument'—rather than see ourselves as called or constituted by it. We like co-ordinates and landmarks. But neither situation is clear-cut. With regard to mindfulness practice, we might recall the story of the Buddhist monk Bodhidharma who challenged a student to bring him the mind he wanted liberating. 'Where are you?' was the implicit question. The student could not meet the challenge, so Bodhidharma claimed to have liberated the student's mind (Ferguson, 2000: 20). Here we might recall Merleau-Ponty's suggestion that words can "teach me my thoughts" (Gordon, 2013: 22) So, far from being seeking, speaking subjects, each of us may, in fact, be something quite different: one who arises and *is spoken*.

Merleau-Ponty

We can explore some of these questions by looking in more depth at the ideas of Merleau-Ponty, a Western philosopher who was explicitly concerned with the world of lived reality and the challenges of language. Although the phenomenological project in which Merleau-Ponty played a part saw itself as experiential, it nevertheless tried to draw out the common features of how the world presents itself to us. Merleau-Ponty himself, though, sought keenly to avoid the fallacy of misplaced concreteness or reification, which is to say he did not treat abstractions or hypothetical constructs as if they were empirically real. In Merleau-Ponty's case, it can also be the suggestion that moments in an interactive process have enduring substantial reality. This is misleading; so he put the accent on such processes rather than on localised noun-things and thereby aimed to eliminate the recalcitrant subject–object dualism of Husserlian phenomenology. Perception is seen as participatory. There is no transcendental ego. He sought an alternative to the prevailing philosophies of consciousness, to bring us back into the body, and to see the body and the world as reaching into one another: to see the mind as embodied and the body in-the-world.

An object is contextual, conditioned, and perspectival. It is not present in opposition to an absence but against an absence that is "its own innermost constitutive possibility" (Dillon, 1991: 122). Meditation can help reveal this 'spaciousness', the matrix of conditioned arising, how perceptions "disintegrate and reform ceaselessly" (Merleau-Ponty, 1962: 38). It can thus also reveal the absolute and independent object as a nonsensical "illusion of rationalist thought" (Dillon, 1991: 123). There are only "focal figures" against horizons. An open horizon means that the "substantiality" of the object "slips away" (Merleau-Ponty, 1962: 70) What Derrida would call 'presence'—any notional essence—"is possible only when in our thinking we forget what we had originally learned in our perceptual experience of the world" (Dillon, 1991: 123) We do well to remember in this connection that mindfulness is itself a form of such remembering. 'Objects' do not have enduring self-nature. When we are not mindful of this, such reification (of perceptual phenomenon into conceptual object) "congeals the whole of existence, as a crystal placed in a solution suddenly crystallizes it" (Merleau-Ponty, 1962: 71).

We ossify experience into permanent structures; we lose our freshness of response; we regulate and homogenise the incorrigibly plural nature of life.

Uncertain Openness

There is here an implicit challenge to Aristotle's laws of thought—those tenets on which rational discourse is based. These can be stated briefly as: something is what it is and is not something else (law of identity); something cannot both be something and not be it (law of non-contradiction); and either a proposition is true or its negation is true (law of excluded middle). For Merleau-Ponty, such precepts of logic are not a priori and self-standing, but "have their origin in something existing outside or prior to them, namely, our pre-logical, perceptual experience of the world" (Dillon, 1991: 120). The result is that such logic is 'de-centred'—and held to be derivative. One might note again in passing that commentaries on mindfulness practice are often full of references to the de-centring of consciousness. In meditation, we come to a realisation that there is a field of consciousness not limited to the controlling focus of ego. That is embodied dharma practice. Whether the copula is the verb 'to be' or the assumed transcendental essence of self, its status is challenged.

For Merleau-Ponty, we infer the notion of essence from perception. Consequently, the certainty of ideas is not the base of the certainty of perception, but it relies on it. This has significant repercussions:

> If logic has its origin in perception, then the 'conditions of possibility' of logic are not themselves 'logical.' Logic itself is not, accordingly, self-grounding; it is not, and cannot be, a *foundational description* (Dillon, 1991: 121).

Our "perceptual experience of the world"—via a process of abstraction in our "idealizing imagination" leads to the notion of identity. This is at bottom nothing other than "a structural characteristic of the *perceptual field*" (ibid: 121). We are thus brought back into our perceptual bodies and the world—and out of the abstractions of rational thought. Loy argues—from a Buddhist perspective, but in strikingly similar language—that we cling to a notion of reified selfhood as an attempt at such self-grounding (1996: 11–12).

Merleau-Ponty's philosophy is a philosophy of ambiguity: we are *not* intelligible, luminous, transparent, universal, univocal, self-same. For Merleau-Ponty, "ambiguity is the essence of human existence, everything we live or think has always several meanings" (1962: 169). This is not a deficiency of consciousness or existence, but, conversely, marks the very richness of life. We are an uncertain openness.

In *Phenomenology of Perception*, Merleau-Ponty (1962) sought a " 'third genus' of corporeal being" (Levin, 1985: 24), beyond both the kind of idealist subjectivism we have seen above, but without resorting to scientific objectivism. This, his early model, was arguably still too Cartesian, and it also missed the "primordial dimensionality of our embodiment...our *pre-ontological* bodily attunement" (ibid: 62). He was more successful in his last book, *The Visible and the Invisible* in his "deconstruction of this rigid subject–object polarity" and of the "egology and objectivity of the body" (1968: 65).

In this later work, the body and the perceived world "form a single system of intentional relations"; in other words, a "double aspect" (Loy, 1988: 95)—and we have already seen how slippery that can be to conceptualise and express. Loy writes: "The body and its sense-organs are objectifications of the ways we tend to thought–condition perceptions" (ibid). It is always worth recalling that the 'mind' is itself a sense organ in early Buddhism (Brazier, 2003: 45)—think: 'mind's eye'; and 'theory'—the modern Western term—comes from *theoria*, meaning a 'way of seeing' in ancient Greek. The split between the sensible and the intelligible is, in such light, not so clear-cut at all. Levin would seem to concur and go a step further—in what is, more accurately, a process without steps: "The body of feeling as we experience it, as we live it, *integrates* what objective thought would divide" (1983: 49). Merleau-Ponty and subsequent theorists of embodiment are certainly aware of how the rational mind can mislead us. It is this thought-conditioning—especially reversion to objectifying thought patterns, differentiations, and impressions (*papañca* e *samskaras* in Buddhist terminology)—that mindfulness, too, seeks to uncover.

Moving into the body tends to move us out of the mind, even if it risks, in so doing, simply relocating a reified self.

The Flesh

Merleau-Ponty developed an ontology of the *flesh*—a term having a very precise meaning for him: we sense and are sensed; or, we are sensate and sensible. From the distinct subject of perception of his earlier work, he moves to a much more intertwined view of our existence in *The Visible and the Invisible* (1968), where flesh stands for everything that is sensible (i.e., that which is sensed). Rather than describing seeing as an act involving a subject who does the seeing, he writes of "visibility, sometimes wandering, sometimes reassembled" (ibid: 254). There are no longer subjects and objects, but a 'fold' in which the sensible reveals itself. We are back to the idea of enfoldedness. And the sensate (i.e., that which senses) reveals itself, too—the process is reversible or, to use one of his key terms, *chiasmatic*.

Touching and being touched are *not*, however, experienced simultaneously: they do not coincide; there is a gap between them. Reflectiveness intrudes: it cannot be sensed in itself and is apprehended as the invisible idea of the visible, an aspect of our incarnation that gives the sensible its depth. Merleau-Ponty compares it to the *memory* of a musical phrase that is *not* real (i.e., sensible), but cannot be *dissociated* from its sensible incarnation.

To summarise: the 'subject' is not the subject of perception as we might ordinarily think, but there *is* a very human reflectiveness associated with sensing that gives it profundity. In spite of naming a gap (*écart*), Merleau-Ponty does not present a dualistic view between mind and body or self and other, for these are, for him, deeply intertwined. Relationships are mutually constitutive: "The world is wholly inside, and I am outside, myself" (1962: 407). There is reversibility and interpenetration.

Embodied subjectivity is never completely located in one pole or other, but at junctions, where the two lines entwine. There is a convergence, as well as a divergence, in a dynamic interaction, and this interdependence is the *flesh*. That the world is not simply an object, as Merleau-Ponty writes in *The Visible and the Invisible*,

> does not mean that there was a fusion or coinciding of me with it: on the contrary, this occurs because a sort of dehiscence opens my body in two, and because between my body looked at and my body looking, my body touched and my body touching, there is overlapping or encroachment, so that we may say that the things pass into us, as well as we into the things (1968: 132).

We exist as this non-dualistic divergence/convergence, and are assured that absolute antinomy between self and world is resisted. Merleau-Ponty frequently invokes ideas of the 'in between' and an 'interworld' in his writing. And, as we have seen, some of his commentators, too, invoke non-duality overtly: "the phenomenal world is ontologically and epistemologically prior to the worlds of subjectivity and objectivity which dualist thought posits as primary reality" (Dillon, 1988: 88).

Mindfulness

For Merleau-Ponty, phenomenology seeks to "return to the world that precedes knowledge, of which knowledge always *speaks*" (Abram, 1997: 36). There is a clear overlap here between the theories of Merleau-Ponty and those of Dōgen. For the latter, the human body participates in the external world. Mind, body, and things of the world "interpenetrate one another without the possibility of a lucid demarcation among them (Olson, 1986: 109). Dōgen's "nondualistic position" is "similar to what Merleau-Ponty calls the flesh" (ibid).

Rather than reflective intentional consciousness, Dōgen moves towards a non-thinking (*hishiryo*) acceptance, which is a "'thinking' of the unthinkable or emptiness", with no abstracted division between body and mind or self and world (Olson, 1986: 110).

Mindfulness is awareness of whatever arises. If we sharpen and broaden our awareness, we become acutely aware of *dukkha* (affliction). But we also become aware that what often underpins *dukkha* is the misappropriation of a reified self, and, moreover, that what is reified can all too easily be deified. We readily seek to become masters of our own universe, inner and outer.

The split between self and world is coarse, but there is usually another, more subtle sense of division between 'I' (in a kinaesthetic or proprioceptive register) and 'me' (as somatic or objective/specular entity—as if looking at oneself in a mirror). This is what Berman calls the basic fault. He argues that "true enlightenment is to really know, really feel, your ontological dilemma, your somatic nature" (1989: 310). The upshot is that "the real goal of a spiritual tradition should not be ascent, but openness, vulnerability, and this does not require great experiences but, on the contrary, very ordinary ones" (ibid: 310). This is not about the quest for some great beyond. It is about realising the birth and death in every moment. The body—in the breath, in its ever-changing feeling-tones, in the ageing process—is less able to maintain an illusion of permanence (i.e., secure, uninterrupted presence).

One can remain in the linguistic realm and suggest such a horizontal reality that is not constantly compromising itself in search of transcendence—that is open to the other and to change. Epstein writes:

> Realisation that self is not reified but a metaphor, mirage or fiction can be disconcerting but according to Buddhist psychology, this understanding is liberating... Difficult emotions such as anger, fear,

and selfish desire are all predicated on this misperception of self. When the representational nature of self is fully appreciated, therefore, these emotions lose their source of inspiration (1996: 154).

Self is another story—the one that underpins all others and thinks it *sees*. But when awareness is alive to the reality of unfolding existence—'self' is itself *seen*.

It is the self, specifically the rationalistic ego, that seeks to dominate with a "territorial logic which is both colonizing and predatory" (Fiumara, 1990: 65), and it is the rationalistic (and rationalising) ego that mindfulness practice can help us investigate. We move from seeing the world through it to seeing through it *tout court*. Instead of constantly and defensively retelling pre-told stories, and *assuming* a relational mutuality or common ground with others, the better route is to encounter the other and create something new. In this regard, mindfulness is of great value. In a sense, true mindfulness makes poets of us all: it allows life in its otherness to come to us without the homogenising filter of self. There is something similar in the work of Merleau-Ponty, in his accent on the "mystery of the familiar" in the "pre-theoretical substrate of experience" (Critchley, 2001: 115).

Unfortunately, the Western application of mindfulness often limits itself to observation of the thought process for the quasi-technological regulation of affect (passions/emotions). Rather than challenging our desire for control, it risks feeding it. One of the main purposes of dharma practice is reaching an understanding of the nature of self as 'empty' (the doctrine of *anatman*): as nothing more (or less) than an aggregate of processes or *skandhas*. One could compare this with Merleau-Ponty's notion of the sedimentation of the *habitual body*, which is contrasted with the living, *present body* (Merleau-Ponty, 1962). The former is the bodily schema that denotes the precognitive familiarity with self and world, but which tends to attenuate freshness of response. One might go further and suggest that we choose the deadness of habit in a fruitless attempt to avoid the life and death in each moment, and, ultimately, physical death. If we are already dead, we do not have to face dying.

When considered reflectively, 'nature' becomes a part of culture. Mindfulness can heal the breach between the mental and the environmental. It can reveal the mental as a conditioned element of the environment (each as a function of the other) after which the distinction too collapses. Through mindfulness practice, we can gradually come to accept our resistances, understand our compulsions, notice what distracts us, see into our delusions and the nature of our conditioning. In the spaciousness of meditation, there is, at the very least, room for knots and vicious circles to loosen. Enfoldedness need not mean entanglement.

The emphasis in dharma practice is on the experiential: it is inner physics rather than metaphysics. This does not mean that it is predicated on escape from fundamental concerns. It means just the opposite: it is an embodied awareness of impermanence and *dukkha*, but one that may reveal how we overlay the pain of existence with our own elaborate suffering. When the 'inner' self is seen as fiction, the 'outer' other can enter awareness. Consciousness becomes less claustrophobic. *Sunyata*, often translated as 'emptiness', can here be understood as 'openness', its etymology suggesting something pregnant with possibility. There is room for surprise. In this sense, too, mindfulness practice is not self-absorbed introspection but ethical engagement. This is where it does overlap with the aims of modern theory: "Deconstruction is not an enclosure in nothingness, but openness towards the other" (Critchley, 1992: 28). All is not wrapped up into a unitary meta-narrative by a unitary self. Plurality and encounter can thrive. Mark Epstein writes:

> It is through the mindfulness practices that Buddhism most clearly complements psychotherapy. The shift from an appetite-based, spatially conceived self preoccupied with a sense of what is lacking to a breath-based, temporally conceived self capable of spontaneity and aliveness is, of course, one that psychotherapy has also come to envision (1996: 145).

Mindfulness is both criticised and praised for its emphasis on the 'now', the quasi-mystical *nunc stans*: 'momentism.' But if difference allows us to see, we might say the same of time which is, after all, simply a measure of change or difference. 'We' do not exist in time, but *as* time, living and dying in each moment. Being *is* time. For Buddhism, this reality of impermanence—*anicca*—is one of the marks of existence. All is flux. On this, too, Merleau-Ponty and Dōgen are in agreement. For the former, the body inhabits time: "Like a work of art that is indistinguishable from the existence that expresses it, and its temporality is indistinguishable from it. In a sense, within my body I am time" (Olson, 1986: 112). For the latter, all things—including us—are manifestations of being-time (*uji*).

If we need to envision ourselves at all it may be better, as Epstein (1996) suggests, to think less in terms of space—of a thing enduring in a specific location—and more in terms of time. It is curious that stories exist in time and are, as such, affirmations of becoming; and yet our stories of ourselves and reality seem so fixed and resistant to change. There is movement in stories—but to preordained ends.

For Aristotle, man is the language-using animal—*zoon logon ekon*. For Merleau-Ponty, man is similarly 'possessed' by language as much as its possessor. He is *in* a world of language just as he is *in* a world of perception. He is not a being who experiences and expresses; he is experiential being and expression.

On the one hand, there is also a playful dimension both in meditation and our interaction with the world. On the other hand, however, language suggests fixed co-ordinates in its depiction of reality, a specific location, and set of conditions. There is often something diagrammatic about it. 'This is how it is', it says. It may denote change but can never keep up with it or fully reflect its complexity. It is often more *le dit* (the words spoken) than *le dire* (the live act of speaking). This may well mean that the less we struggle to define and denote self/world, the more philosophical language—the medium of definition and denotation—will. The less we seek to hold our place, the more written words may lose their halo and appear as placeholders—*even* those at the edge, reaching beyond themselves.

Grammatically, 'self' is a noun and, more realistically, a verb. Mindfulness (another noun) and some of our more insightful theorists (other selves) can help us see this.

Yet no amount of words can quite catch it and do it, or us, justice.

References

Abram, D. (1997) *The Spell of the Sensuous* (London: Vintage).
Bateson, G. (2000) *Steps to an Ecology of Mind: Collected Essays in Anthropology, Psychiatry, Evolution, and Epistemology* (Chicago, IL: University of Chicago Press).
Berman, M. (1989) *Coming to Our Senses* (London: Unwin Hyman).
Brazier, C. (2003) *Buddhist Psychology* (London: Robinson).
Critchley, S. (1992) *The Ethics of Deconstruction* (Oxford: Blackwell).
Critchley, S. (2001) *Continental Philosophy* (Oxford: Oxford University Press).
Dillon, M. C. (1988) *Merleau-Ponty's Ontology* (Evanston, IL: Northwestern University Press).
Dillon, M. C. (ed.) (1991) *Merleau-Ponty Vivant* (Albany, NY: SUNY Press).
Epstein, M. (1996) *Thoughts Without a Thinker* (London: Duckworth).
Gordon, P. (2013) 'A Philosophy of Wonder,' *Therapy Today*, February, 20–2.
Ferguson, A. (2000) *Zen's Chinese Heritage* (Boston, MA: Wisdom Publications).
Fiumara, G. C. (1990) *The Other Side of Language – A Philosophy of Listening* (London: Routledge).

Flemons, D. G. (1991) *Completing Distinctions* (Boston, MA: Shambala).

Hanh, T. N. (1975) *The Miracle of Mindfulness* (Boston, MA: Beacon Press).

Honderich, T. (ed.) (1995) *Oxford Companion to Philosophy* (Oxford: Oxford University Press).

Kabat-Zinn, J. (1994) *Wherever You Go, There You Are: Mindfulness Meditation in Everyday Life* (New York: Hyperion).

Lawson, H. (1985) *Reflexivity* (London: Hutchinson).

Levin, D. M. (1985) *The Body's Recollection of Being* (London: Routledge).

Loy, D. (1988) *Nonduality* (New York: Humanity Books).

Loy, D. (1996) *Lack and Transcendence: The Problem of Death and Life in Psychotherapy, Existentialism, and Buddhism* (New York: Humanity Books).

Merleau-Ponty, M. (1962) *Phenomenology of Perception* (London: Routledge).

Merleau-Ponty, M. (1968) *The Visible and the Invisible* (Evanston, IL: Northwestern University Press).

Olson, C. (1986) 'The Human Body as a Boundary Symbol: a Comparison of Merleau-Ponty and Dōgen,' *Philosophy East and West*, 36, 2.

Rorty, R. (1989) *Contingency, Irony, and Solidarity* (Oxford and New York: Cambridge University Press).

Wang, Y. (2001) 'Liberating Oneself from the Absolutized Boundary of Language: a Liminological Approach to the Interplay of Speech and Silence in Chan Buddhism,' *Philosophy East and West*, 51, 1.

Watts, A. (1975) *Psychotherapy East and West* (New York: Vintage).

Wittgenstein, L. (1972) *On Certainty* (London: Harper Perennial).

10
Clinical Mindfulness, Meta-perspective, and True Nature

Dheeresh Turnbull

Introduction

I would be reluctant to say anything at all about the relation between mindfulness and therapy if I had not had some varied experience on the receiving end of both as student and client/patient, in addition to working as a cognitive–behavioural therapist and leading eight-week mindfulness-based stress reduction (MBSR) groups.

I would like to suggest that there are five different paths of therapeutic change within the individual, each with potential pitfalls.

1. *Starting With Emotion/Body*. Working with emotions directly is difficult because one (client or therapist) can be 'in one's head' and mistake an emotion for a thought, or vice versa. However, if you start with body sensation, and use that to access the emotion, then you are on firmer ground (as thoughts by themselves don't have associated body sensations). The client may then have a profound experience or release. This may feel good at the time, but will, perhaps, have little long-term effect unless the insight of what needs to change (to prevent the unhealthy pattern re-establishing itself) is drawn out. And while sometimes you simply need to get stuff 'off your chest', the body emotion version can descend into toothpaste-tube therapy ('all we've got to do is squeeze it out').

2. *Starting With Thought*. This is the style of most cognitive–behavioural therapy (CBT). The main advantage is that one can learn to stand back from one's thoughts (easier than with feelings, for example). And if the thought changes, sometimes the emotion will also change. Unfortunately, one can fall into the hole of 'right answer CBT' where the person can see a theoretically healthier way of looking at their problem, but because the emotion or heart isn't touched,

feelings don't change and neither does behaviour. John Teasdale (Teasdale and Barnard, 1993; Teasdale, 1996) talks about the need to access 'implicational' (heart-) mind for therapy to be effective; when only 'propositional' (logical-) mind is affected, then nothing really happens...

3. *Starting Interpersonally*. This, combined to a greater or lesser extent with point 1 above, is the style of much counselling and psychotherapy work. While, of course, this helps us to see that no man (or woman) is an island, and the consulting room can become a ready-made laboratory to experiment interpersonally, it can be polluted by the therapist unwittingly bringing their own 'stuff' to the consulting room, either in terms of unresolved personal material, or therapeutic axes to grind. The likelihood of this happening is, in my opinion, inversely proportional to the degree of agreed structure in the session.

4. *Starting With Behaviour*. On one level, this can be very effective, for example as in exposure and response prevention with obsessive compulsive disorder. Padmal de Silva (Kwee, 1990) was fond of showing how various behaviour therapy (BT) techniques were a favourite of the Buddha. However, one needs to know which behaviour needs to change, and associated thoughts and emotions need also to be tracked so that one doesn't become a dissociated robot! I would suggest that the BT approach can obviously be useful for symptom reduction, but sometimes the symptoms are an expression of something else in the thought-and-feeling department, and if this is not addressed, they may recur in the same, or different, form.

5. *Starting With Awareness*. This is the meditation route. For some people, the conventional sitting-down version of this can be too much to begin with—the mind contents just feel too overwhelming and distressing, although Marsha Linehan (1993) has shown how focused present-centred awareness can be a way of *staying with* difficult emotions, for example typically for those with a diagnosis of borderline personality disorder. The key questions (to my mind) are (a) whether awareness by itself can ever be enough, and (b) whether one can sustain the changes once one leaves the meditation environment. Jack Kornfield (2000) has documented what can go wrong in that area. In relation to the former, I would suggest that many students have used meditation as a form of experiential avoidance. Yet it is practically a truism to say that one has to develop an awareness of a problem in order to begin to address it. Which leads us neatly to the next section.

What is Mindfulness?

The current favoured description of mindfulness in clinical circles is the one that appears in *The Mindful Way through Depression*: "The awareness that comes from paying attention without judgement in the present moment to things as they are" (Williams et al., 2007: 47). While this is a wonderful description, I think it is also worth reminding ourselves that the literal meaning of the word *sati* (Pali), or *smṛti* (Sanskrit), usually translated by the English word 'mindfulness' actually means 'remembered' (originally, in Hinduism, as opposed to *shruti*, 'revealed'). Of course, that is already open to a number of interpretations, one of which might be that we are remembering to remember—bringing ourselves back into the present, so to speak. Or, perhaps, in that very concept there is the germ of an understanding, an acceptance that we have *forgotten who we really are*. When we begin to realise that we have forgotten, then we can start to do something about it. In a way, all therapeutic and spiritual/meditational disciplines could be seen as different versions of that task.

Meta-perspective

The concept of *meta-perspective* gives us a way of analysing these different disciplines and potentially of aiding clinicians in selecting the right balance of interventions for themselves and those they seek to help. In addition, this concept may partly lead us to a different overview, which can help us to transcend at least some of the apparent contradictions between the various styles and methods of therapy listed above.

What is 'meta-perspective'? It is the *position* from which we view our mind-contents—our psycho-therapeutic stance on ourselves. There are, in my view, two major types of meta-perspective, which I call *horizontal* and *vertical*.

Horizontal meta-perspective is the position most commonly taken by CBT and also by mindfulness-based techniques like MBSR, mindfulness-based cognitive therapy, and acceptance and commitment therapy (ACT). It is where we break down our mind contents into a variety of (interactive) components: thoughts, feelings/emotions, body sensations, and behaviours, for example. I call it *horizontal* on the analogy of a workbench: you have the parts all laid out, and then perhaps wire them up to each other in different combinations to see what happens. We examine the interaction between the different components, and then we either seek to change one or more components (thought and behaviour are the most common), or simply to distance ourselves from that component: 'it's just a thought', we might say.

Even if, as in CBT, we start out by substituting one thought for another, in the end what one is looking to cultivate is detachment or '*stand-back-ability*' as one realises the relative and sometimes arbitrary nature of the thought or feeling. As we learn to stand back, sometimes we can realise that what we thought of as a 'real-world' problem turns out to be a psychological problem, as is often the case in panic disorder (PD) or obsessive compulsive disorder (OCD).

For example, the CBT approach to the treatment of PD, where sometimes people believe they are going to have a heart attack, is to encourage the awareness that the problem is not that 'I am going to have a heart attack', but that 'I am *afraid that* I am going to have a heart attack' because of a catastrophic misinterpretation of bodily sensations (Clark, 1988, 1996) This is not so much an alternative cognition as a shift in view, or logical level, or ... *meta-perspective*. Similarly, in contamination OCD, the problem is not actually that the sufferer is contaminated, but that they *feel* contaminated. They have, as it were, an over-sensitive 'yuck-o-meter', which has been triggered by association.

As sufferers from these, and other, conditions *learn to mistrust* their automatic thinking minds or their intrusive thoughts and sensations, then they can step back from being hooked up in the contents and can see better what is going on, and thus break free from being dominated by their symptoms. While this approach can be tremendously helpful, there are sometimes glitches in treatment, where, even though people *know* that they are not going to have a heart attack and that it is 'only' panic, they go on having panic attacks.

The recurrence of panic is, in my opinion, to be attributed to the fact that only half the question has been answered. If we accept that these sensations are a 'catastrophic misinterpretation of bodily sensation', that only gets us halfway. The other part of the question is, "What *are* the body sensations trying to tell me?"

Vertical meta-perspective is when another way of looking at our 'stuff' becomes helpful. Where horizontal meta-perspective looks at gaining detachment from our components, by seeing them as components in interaction (rather than 'me' or 'the truth'), vertical meta-perspective also looks at parts, but in the sense of *sub-personalities*. This approach seeks to hear from the parts, each of them endowed with its own thoughts, feelings, body sensations, and associated behavioural tendencies. So, for example, someone having a panic attack was asked by the therapist to breathe into the sensations. She burst into tears, "It's my mother", she said, "I'm having such a hard time with her at the moment." "That must be upsetting", the therapist commented. And after a little while sympathising about her relationship with the mother, "By the way, what happened to the panic sensations?", "Oh, they've gone" she said...

My contention is that the body sensations were informing her of an unacknowledged threat. The alarm system that is panic was trying to get her attention. A purely horizontal approach here would not have been effective. The two parts, which *both needed to be heard*, were panic and relationship-with-mother. Once relationship-with-mother had been allowed to come to the surface, panic disappeared because its job was done.

While horizontal meta-perspective cultivates *detachment*, vertical meta-perspective cultivates *enquiry*. And while clinical mindfulness tends only to emphasise the horizontal, more traditional, Buddhist meditation training also brings in the vertical standpoint. My first Buddhist teacher introduced me to the five hindrances: lust; ill-will; sloth and torpor; restlessness and worry; and doubt. These are parts— 'sub-personalities'—not components. However, this is where an understanding of the multifaceted nature of self is vital. People will only feel safe digging into particular parts if they realise that whatever it is they're uncovering, it is *not the whole story*. If I know that even the most abject and profound despair is *not the whole of me*, it becomes safe for me to feel it.

While techniques based on horizontal meta-perspective can be very helpful for certain conditions, and while the detachment cultivated is almost always a pre-requisite for effective change, it may not always be enough. There may be parts (programmes, sub-personalities, or other aspects or voices) that need to be heard in order for the problems to be either resolved or at least accepted. This requires the adoption of techniques based on vertical meta-perspective.

Programmes and Selves

If we are thinking about meditation/mindfulness in relation to therapeutic change, and we accept that simply working horizontally, although useful, may not always be enough, and may sometimes even be a way of avoiding one's emotional difficulties, then we need to look at what the different sorts of little 'I's' are that we may need to uncover and work with. That will include a willingness to accept that some of them may not be changeable, but simply need to be acknowledged. These little 'Is' can be thought of as programmes which mostly arose in response to particular situations, some of which pre-dated the species, never mind the birth or even the conception of the individual.

Levels of Programming

I suggest we can identify five levels of programming: *prehistoric*, which, for convenience, we can sub-divide into three (reptilian and paleo-mammalian; simian; and cave-man); *human genetic*; *local cultural*; *perinatal*; and *personal historical*. The earlier parts are obviously built in to our structure. However, although people used to think that brain structure was totally fixed by adulthood, we now know that neuro-plasticity is a fact (Schwartz and Begley, 2002; Hanson and Mendius, 2009). Similarly, we should not assume that these phylogenetically earlier parts are 'dead', cannot have a voice, or do not have something to say (Turnbull, 2013). We should also not assume that these prehistoric parts are identically formed in different individuals. I would suggest, for example, that different genetic memories may be responsible for differing reactions to spiders or snakes.

In some of these programmes we don't really know what is alterable, even assuming that this were desirable. But in acknowledging and sometimes hearing from the different levels, we can at least understand their influence and sometimes wishes. Again, a good 'vertical' technique may be able to help us access most, if not all, of these to find out what's getting 'fired up' in any disturbance.

What are good vertical techniques? My experience is inevitably limited, but a working definition could be *anything eliciting the voice of a particular part without traumatising the individual in the process*. The most well-known may be the empty chair technique from Gestalt Therapy (Perls, 1969). Transactional Analysis is also relevant (Berne 1964/2010), as is imagery re-scripting in cognitive (Hackmann et al., 2011) or schema therapy (McGinn and Young, 1996). The last decade or so has seen the arrival of the big mind process from D. Genpo Merzel (2007), a development of Hal and Sidra Stone's voice dialogue (1989), which incorporates a spiritual, boundless awareness.

Goal-setting and 'True Nature'

What are we trying to do in (potentially) awakening all these voices? Naturally, the therapist should be guided primarily by the wishes of the client. But there are times where it may be helpful to point out the odd 'home truth': for example, if you have been off work with stress repeatedly in the last year, should we really be keeping unquestioningly to the goal of getting back to work?

This brings us to the concept of 'true nature.' A favourite question in ACT is "What do you want to have written on your tombstone?", which we could paraphrase as "Are you living in line with what is really an expression of who you are?" This might be applied to work, or relationships, or anything else important to the client. Of course, this is predicated on the idea that the person knows who they really are, when, in fact, they may not even have asked the question (yet).

Self, no Self, and True Self

Here, I think, we have arrived at the heart of the matter. In Buddhism, the three marks of conditioned existence are unsatisfactoriness ('suffering': *dukkha* in Pali); temporariness (*anicca*), and no-self (*anatta*). I don't think that 'no-self' automatically means that people in the Buddha's time were all suffering from what we might today call an 'identity crisis.' On the contrary, in what was perhaps a less complicated age, I suspect most people did not struggle with the 'What am I here for?' question, and the issue of low self-esteem was probably as foreign to them as it was (apparently) to the Dalai Lama when he first encountered it among Western meditation teachers. I don't, however, mean to imply life was necessarily better then.

True Nature

With the confusing range of expectations and competing priorities that the modern world presents us with, it is not surprising that we struggle. Before we go any further, it is important to distinguish two meanings of the term 'true nature.' The first, and the traditional Zen understanding of 'true nature' or 'true self', is to come to a full, experiential awareness of 'no-self' or 'no-mind.' We are ultimately one with the universe and not separate. And whoever/however we are, this does not change.

As Charlotte Joko Beck has it: "true self—call it the infinite energy potential—knows no separation. True self forms into different shapes but essentially it remains one self, one energy potential" (1997: 92). This is our 'true nature' in the Zen sense. If we are very fortunate, we may discover a teacher who will lead us to a taste of this or more. Mindfulness is definitely helpful in coming to our true nature in this sense, and, one could argue, this is the purpose for which mindfulness was originally devised. But experiences of enlightenment or liberation will not solve all our problems of being-in-the-world, although they may help us remain sanguine when things go wrong.

To use a well-worn metaphor, we are the ocean: we are all sea-water, that's what we're made of, and that's what we revert to at the end of our individual existence. This is the truth of no-self. But each wave is unique, and temporary, and has its own never-to-be repeated pattern and combination of molecules: this is the truth of self. In human terms, that means we are different, relatively, from each other, and not just in the way we present ourselves.

Of course, the process of discovering who one is—what one is built for if you like—is a complementary *but different* process to that of discovering that one is not separate from the whole.

Different Buddha-minds

Buddhism underwent a transformation with the growth of the Mahayana school, which rejected the ideal of individual enlightenment in favour of endeavouring to save all sentient beings. In this new doctrine, there arose the idea of the three bodies of the Buddha (Williams, 1989): the Dharmakāya, which is the boundless infinite, empty yet all-inclusive; the *Sambhogakāya*, which is the 'bliss-body'—the glorious manifestation of Buddhahood; and the *Nirmanakāya*, which is the ordinary human body which Gautama, who came to be known as Siddhartha, and later 'the Buddha', was born into. Given that, at least according to most versions, we all have what it takes to be Buddha, I think we can take these ideas and apply them to ourselves and, in doing so, it will hopefully clarify further the subject at hand.

Nirvana, or enlightenment, is one of the very few phenomena described as 'unconditioned' in Buddhist writings. Space is another. The quest for enlightenment was what drove most practitioners of Buddhist (and other sorts of) meditation. The goal was liberation from suffering. The conventional track was probably (though not always) a mixture of *samatha* (calm) and *vipassana* (insight) meditation. Clinical mindfulness is mostly an offshoot of the latter. However one went about it, the goal was to penetrate through the illusion of the world-separated-into-self-and-not-self, with (if successful) an outcome of unbounded wisdom and compassion, that is, an experience of being the ocean (to use our previous metaphor). In terms of the doctrine of the three bodies, this is the realisation of the Dharmakāya, the ultimate, which transcends all suffering: true nature in the Zen sense.

However, the confusion between the realisation of emptiness and effective functioning in the world has led various spiritual teachers to think that if they've had a taste of the Absolute, particularly a strong and profound taste, that means they've got to be 'sorted' all the time, never feel any 'negative' emotions, and so on, and give their students top-quality advice on whom to marry, how to vote, what to do with difficult emotions, and so on.

Clinical mindfulness, however, is employed, quite reasonably, for therapeutic purposes. It is not about realising the Dharmakāya but about working more efficiently with the Nirmanakāya: our body in the world. Of course, from time to time, students may have blissful experiences (Sambhogakāya), and even a taste of emptiness (Dharmakāya), but this is, to coin a phrase, more about what happens when you don't sweat the small stuff. Just learning to be in the present more, in the body more, appreciative of every little thing (whether we like it or not), is tremendously therapeutic, and increases our quality of life and our interactions. But from a more traditional Buddhist perspective, it is just the beginning.

From a therapeutic perspective, if we only work horizontally, we don't really address the question of emotional avoidance in our lives—although difficult stuff will certainly come up when we're sitting in meditation.

To summarise: psychologists have happily stumbled upon mindfulness techniques that facilitate 'stand-back-ability' from our mind contents, thus enabling us to stay with difficult emotions, while enhancing our appreciation of life. This has served well in helping people in various states of physically- and mentally-generated distress. Meanwhile, traditional spiritual teachers of meditation have kept up the tradition of helping students to have a taste of the infinite, or Dharmakāya, but have sometimes, unfortunately, been cast in the role of therapist, for which they have not been trained.

True Nature Revisited

What may complement this rather confused state of affairs is to separate out the therapeutic from the spiritual, at least so that we know what we're doing when we're doing it. It is a happy accident that mindfulness is useful, for example in preventing relapse in recurrent depression.

Perhaps there are some other techniques that might, if adopted, reduce the likelihood of the onset of depression in the first place. Perhaps we need to think again about *true nature*, but less in an absolute, Dharmakāya kind of way and more in a relative, *Prakriti* (nature) kind of way. Prakriti, like many Sanskrit technical terms, is used by different schools in different ways. In one Shamanic tradition, the *Shuh Shuh Guh*, it means 'true nature': who we really are, as in what we're built for when we arrive on the planet. So—*given* that we're all ocean—what *kind of a wave* am I/was I meant to be (before all the traumas, conditioning and weight of different expectations got layered on top)?

To find this out is a different process from simply learning to stand back (horizontal), although the ability to do that is to some extent a pre-requisite—like 'access concentration' in mindfulness, one needs a certain *stillness* just to be able to look. It is also a different process from 'becoming one with' in the Zen sense.

Sometimes psychotherapy, particularly of a 'vertical' kind, can help us towards a sense of true nature in this individual sense. But in remaining within the boundaries of what has conventionally been thought of as the self, we are cut off from much information. An alternative, broader view (which in many ways parallels the Big Mind process already referred to) can be found in shamanic traditions.

One such shamanic version of this process—the 'Journey to Self'—involves letting go of the past; uncovering and releasing shadows (which we could call 'disowned' voices); learning to distinguish between those selves that are part of one's 'Prakriti' and those which are conditioned add-ons (and releasing those), and allowing one's dreams and wishes—Prakriti's dreams and wishes—to come to the surface and be realised.

A set of tools of the kind one learns on such a journey helps complement clinical mindfulness so that we do not use mindfulness, psychotherapy, or any other techniques unwittingly to push *against* the flow of our nature, and helps us be with our emotions in a way that honours them appropriately. Additionally, it gives us a much more stable base from which to embark on the 'journey to the other shore' if so wished. After all, Nirmanakaya means transformation-body.

Conclusion

Through the ideas of meta-perspective (horizontal and vertical) and two different conceptions of true nature, we have explored two overlapping processes: one, the quest for enlightenment or liberation from suffering, and two, the 'journey to self'—how to live more fully and more easily in the world and go some way to fulfilling one's potential. We have identified that a degree of stillness or 'access concentration' and 'stand-back-ability', such as cultivated in mindfulness meditation, is necessary for both endeavours.

However, learning to stand back from mind contents generally, and even being able to become one with (or realise that one is already one with) 'the ocean', may not in itself be sufficient to live a helpful/productive/satisfying life-in-the-world—learning to be the kind of wave you really are. By distinguishing the concerns of the Nirmanakāya from those of the Dharmakāya, we can be clear which enterprise we are involved in, and hopefully be successful in both. Of course, the Nirmanakāya means transformation body. Whether we interpret that in the traditional Mahayana fashion, that is, that the apparent physicality of the Buddha was, in fact, simply a conjuring trick, or, more kindly, as skilful means enabling us lowly humans to wake up to enlightenment; or whether we say, in a rather less religious mode, that the best function of this bodily existence is to transform itself into the best and most awake kind of being it can possibly be—I leave the choice to the reader.

Is mindfulness intrinsically therapeutic? I would say yes and no. Yes, because it makes us aware of our components (horizontal) and their processing, or which parts (vertical) have become activated. Eventually, one may tire of repeating the seemingly endless patterns clearly seen through meditation. No, because its original tendency is toward accessing Sambhogakāya (bliss) and Dharmakāya (emptiness), whereas therapy is primarily about transforming Nirmanakāya (body-in-the-world)—although the latter may often be a prerequisite for working with the other two.

This is not in any way to decry or belittle the therapeutic effects undoubtedly felt by many practitioners of clinical mindfulness. It is simply to point out that when we use a tool for something other than that for which it was already intended, we may need to complement it with something else from the infinitely varied toolbox that is human spiritual/therapeutic practice.

References

Beck, C. J. (1997) *Everyday Zen: Love and Work* (London: Thorsons, Harper Collins).

Berne, E. (1964/2010) *Games People Play: The Psychology of Human Relationships* (Harmondsworth: Penguin).

Clark, D. M. (1988) 'A Cognitive Model of Panic', in Rachman, S. and Maser, J. (eds) *Panic: Psychological Perspectives*, pp. 71–90 (Hillsdale, NJ: Erlbaum).

Clark, D. M. (1996) 'Panic Disorder: From Theory to Therapy', in Salkovskis, P. (ed.) *Frontiers of Cognitive Therapy*, pp. 318–44 (New York: Guilford).

Hackmann, A., Bennett-Levy, J. and Holmes, E. A. (2011) *Oxford Guide to Imagery in Cognitive Therapy* (Oxford: Oxford University Press).

Hanson, R. and Mendius, R. (2009) *Buddha's Brain: The Practical Neuroscience of Happiness, Love and Wisdom* (Oakland, CA: New Harbinger Publications).

Kornfield, J. (2000) *After the Ecstasy, the Laundry* (London: Rider).

Kwee, M. G. T. (1990) (ed.) *Psychotherapy, Meditation and Health: A Cognitive-behavioural Perspective* (London/The Hague: East-West Publications).

Linehan, M. (1993) *Cognitive-behavioral Treatment of Borderline Personality Disorder* (New York: Guilford Press).

McGinn, L. K. and Young, J. E. (1996) 'Schema Focused Therapy', in Salkovskis, P. (ed.) *Frontiers of Cognitive Therapy*, pp. 182–207 (New York: Guilford).

Merzel, D. G. (2007) *Big Mind, Big Heart: Finding Your Way* (Salt Lake City, UT: Big Mind Publishing).

Perls, F. S. (1969) *Gestalt Therapy Verbatim* (Lafayette, CA: Real People Press).

Schwartz, J. M. and Begley, S. (2002) *The Mind & The Brain: Neuroplasticity and the Power of Mental Force* (New York: Regan/Harper Collins).

Stone, H. and Stone, S. (1989) *Embracing our Selves: the Voice Dialogue Manual* (Oakland, CA: Nataraj).

Teasdale, J. D. (1996) 'Clinically Relevant Theory: Integrating Clinical Insight with Cognitive Science', in Salkowski, P. M. (ed.) *Frontiers of Cognitive Therapy*, pp. 26–47 (New York: Guildford Press).

Teasdale, J. D. and Barnard, P. J. (1993) *Affect, Cognition and Change: Re-modelling Depressive Thought* (Hove: Lawrence Erlbaum).

Turnbull, D. (2013) *Learning to Play Your Mind: The CBT-pot* (Brighton: Penpress).

Williams, P. (1989) *Mahayana Buddhism: The Doctrinal Foundations* (London: Routledge).

Williams, M, Teasdale, J., Segal, Z. and Kabat-Zinn, J (2007) *The Mindful Way through Depression: Freeing Yourself from Chronic Unhappiness* (New York: Guilford Press).

11
The Value of Meditative States of Mind in the Therapist

Monica Lanyado

Introduction

As the world grows smaller with the impact of cheaper travel and the Internet opening up curiosity and exploration of ways of living across the globe, ideas from many different cultures are cross-fertilizing. This is happening in ways that are interesting, as well as worrying; deep, as well as superficial; creative, as well as destructive. The buzz of information can be overwhelming, and the resultant living experience can end up being a muddled multitude of fragmented knowledge insufficiently digested or integrated. We are in the midst of such a significant technological revolution that it is often hard to tell the wood from the trees; to discern what is helpful and worthwhile, and what is a distraction from the path we are trying to travel in life.

In drawing attention to 'new perspectives' on Buddhism and psychology, this volume attempts to reflect on where we are now in thinking about this particular East–West dialogue in the light of the popularity of the idea of 'mindfulness' and its integration into evidence-based psychological treatments. In his fascinating book *The Master and His Emissary*, McGilchrist argues that rather than this being a dialogue, it is a power struggle between very different ways of experiencing the world—ways that are embedded in our brain structure and have played a vital role in the development of worldwide cultures. He writes:

> My thesis is that for us as human beings there are two fundamentally opposed realities, two different modes of experience; that each is of ultimate importance in bringing about the recognizably human world; and that their difference is rooted in the bi-hemispherical structure of the brain. It follows that the two hemispheres need to

co-operate, but I believe that they are in fact involved in a sort of power struggle, and that this explains many aspects of contemporary Western culture (2009: 3).

This 'power struggle' is very alive in the arguments for and against the supremacy of scientific knowledge and methodology over more qualitative or intuitive modes of knowledge. In crude terms, science is portrayed as having certainty in its answers to the questions it poses for itself, whilst philosophy or qualitative approaches of investigation are more able to cope with uncertainty. In reality, scientific knowledge is constantly evolving and is not certain at all. There can be a fierce conflict between knowledge as gained in a scientific way, and wisdom as gained in a more holistic way—presumably from McGilchrist's point of view epitomizing the knowledge-seeking left hemisphere in a power struggle with the wisdom-seeking right one. What follows can be thought of in the context of this interesting thesis.

This chapter offers some ideas from a particular viewpoint within this discussion; broadening ideas about mindfulness to ideas about meditative states of mind in general, and linking these states of mind to what happens between a psychotherapist and her/his patients that enables some recovery or healing to take place. The context is from within the psychoanalytic tradition and, in particular, work with children and young people who have been so seriously traumatized and abused that they have been removed from their birth families and placed for adoption, as was the patient whom I discuss in more detail.

Until fairly recently, possibly the last five to ten years, it has been unusual for psychoanalytic practitioners who are regular meditators to talk or write about how their meditative practice and experience relate to what goes on in the therapy room. An increasing number of psychoanalytic clinicians are now sharing their experiences about their often longstanding meditative practice and the significant ways in which this contributes to their clinical practice, and their way-of-being in the consulting room (Coltart, 1992, 1993, 1996; Epstein, 1995, 2006; Parsons, 2000, 2006; Black, 2006, 2011; Rubin, 2006; Eigen, 2008).

The ideas that follow draw on the writings and experiences of these psychoanalytic practitioners who practice meditation as a regular part of their lives, so much so that it is an integral part of who they are. This relates to what is experienced by the patient as the psychotherapist's authenticity and the psychotherapist's 'presence' when with the patient (Lanyado, 2004). All the psychoanalysts listed above are highly respected clinicians, presumably well psychoanalyzed during, and possibly after, their training, and they clearly do not feel that their meditative practice compromises their psychoanalytic practice and insight. They write, with some caution, about how these two disciplines can enhance each other and, in McGilchrist's terms, 'co-operate' with each other.

In the context of this chapter, the philosophical, spiritual, or religious thinking around the practice of meditation is not so much the issue as the meditative state of mind itself. The publication of a collection of papers by highly respected psychoanalysts, *Psychoanalysis and Religion in the 21st Century: Competitors or Collaborators?* (Black, 2006), from within the library of psychoanalysis series, suggests that discussions about religion, meditation, and spiritual matters are becoming more mainstream within psychoanalysis. Prior to this, there were a number of other thought-provoking publications that contributed to this field and which could possibly be thought of as contributing to the critical mass of writing that was reached with Black's publication (Coltart, 1992, 1993, 1996; Symington, 1994; Epstein, 1995; Molino, 1998; Parsons, 2000). Black's more recent book, *Why Things Matter: The Place of Values in Science, Psychoanalysis and Religion* (2011) develops his ideas, which he describes as having had a gestation period of fifteen years.

From my own experience, it has intrigued me that whenever I have written psychoanalytic papers and given talks that have included ideas about meditation, colleagues whom I might have known for years but did not know they were meditators like myself, have commented that they have only more recently felt that they could speak in psychoanalytic circles about how important their meditation practice is to them personally and professionally. Speaking more openly about this with colleagues has almost felt like a kind of 'coming out.' In the past, Freudian psychoanalysis has taken a reductive view of spiritual or religious beliefs and observances, interpreting them in terms of family relationships, for example the search for an omnipotent father figure (Freud, 1939). Jungians have always respected and included the spiritual aspects of life in their thinking. The unease that many psychoanalytically trained therapists and psychoanalysts have experienced has lead to the masking or hesitancy in using an important aspect of their true self, in the way in which they relate to their patients and colleagues. For many, it has felt odd to keep these two important aspects of who they are separate in their work, but not in their private worlds, particularly when they are often aware of how significantly their meditation practice helps them to survive, think about, and contain their patients' painful and turbulent emotions. It is much easier today than it was even five years ago to make these connections. In the UK there is now a growing network of those interested in exploring the links between their meditative and clinical practice, in experiential, as well as more theoretical, ways.

Why has it been so difficult for psychoanalytic thinkers to bring these ideas into the psychoanalytic arena? Several psychoanalytic writers, for whom meditation and a spiritual life are clearly important, nevertheless caution about the ways in which meditation can be used defensively or in an idealized way rather than creatively, presumably responding to the concerns of the profession. For example Coltart, who has written extensively about what she regards as the "harmonious, mutually enlightening and potentiating" effects of harnessing psychoanalysis and the practice of Buddhism (1996: 128), writes in the same chapter about

> unfortunate cases where meditation has been poorly taught by an inexperienced amateur to someone whose mental health is by no means sound in the first instance but who is led by enthusiasm or sentiment into a territory he had better been strictly warned off. This kind of breakdown, of which I have seen at least three cases, should provide a strong warning against treating meditation as if it were some sort of alternative health gimmick: there has grown up an unfortunate tendency towards this in the West" (1996: 135).

Coltart was writing in the 1990s, before mindfulness-based stress reduction (MBSR), combined with cognitive–behavioral therapy, became an established part of psychological therapies in the UK Public Health System (Kabat-Zinn, 1990; Segal et al., 2002). Her unease about how meditation can be misguidedly used in therapy is related to important issues of diagnosis, and which kind of treatment best suits which kind of diagnosed mental health problem. Currently, it is, of course, enormously tempting, because of severe constraints on public spending, to use briefer psychological treatments that rely on specific techniques such as MBSR practice, in the hope that they will be sufficient for many patients. This grows from the requirement for evidence-based clinical practice within the public sector (the National Health Service in the UK).

However, research on more complex kinds of psychological treatments, such as psychoanalytic psychotherapy, is more difficult to develop because it needs to be more subtle, as well as multi-dimensional. It does not lend itself so well to the kind of measurement and research that is currently available, plus, as a treatment, it is used in much more complex cases in the first place. Again, we see the struggle between knowledge and wisdom ('left' and 'right' brain in McGilchrist's thesis);

that is, what can be 'measured' (although often not nearly as accurately as we might like to think) and what can be observed and experienced by other human beings carefully trained in psychotherapeutic practice.

In addition, one must also bear in mind that it is because of the strain on public health services that only the most severe cases make it through the consulting room door, and often after a long wait. This has, unfortunately, added to the complexity of the problems.

Mindfulness techniques may, nevertheless, be helpful when a lot of recovery has taken place using deeper psychotherapeutic treatments. In the private mental health sector, difficulties may sometimes be addressed before they have grown into a very complex problem and mindfulness-related techniques might be more helpful here. Certainly, many people who are basically emotionally well-adjusted, but suffering from the stresses of ordinary twenty-first century living, can benefit a great deal from the kind of self-help or short courses that use MBSR practices. They can, if they then wish to, develop these mindfulness techniques further by deepening their meditative practice with meditation teachers, and it is here that there is a potential for their practice to lead to the growth of compassion, lowering of the ego, and a positive form of detachment—all arguably very positive forces within the inner world and in relationships. Using mindfulness practice, in the ways promoted by Kabat-Zinn, has never been advocated as an alternative for meditation itself. It is an application of a useful technique from Buddhism for Westerners, but not a substitute for it.

There is another way in which meditation has an impact on psychotherapeutic work. This is when the psychotherapist has a well established meditation practice that introduces her/his meditative state of mind into the therapeutic relationship. This state of mind can then contribute to what takes place in the room between the patient and therapist, in the here and now. Coltart, who was a practicing Buddhist until the end of her life, puts this succinctly:

> The discipline of meditation practice enhances the discipline of one's own contribution to an analytic session which sometimes is, in fact, almost indistinguishable from a form of meditation (1992: 174).

She also tried to clarify, in a helpful way, what is meant by 'meditation' in a broader sense, noting that there are many kinds of meditative practice, all seeking, it could be argued, to attain a similar state of mind in the meditator. To quote Coltart again, these differing meditation practices are designed to clear the mind and open it to self-knowing, truth and understanding; worrying and constant thinking are laid aside, and a kind of empty, alert stillness is aimed for (1993: 113).

It is also helpful to note the use of the idea of 'practice', which is as central to meditation as it is to all kinds of therapeutic work. The word 'practice' indicates a commitment to repeating and learning through experience. The Concise Oxford English Dictionary (1990) defines 'practice' as 'repeated exercise in an activity requiring the development of a skill', and 'action or execution as opposed to theory.' There is no long-term goal other than to improve at whatever is being practiced—be it the piano, football, meditation, or psychoanalytic work. Depending on where and how the meditator is learning to meditate, and who their teacher is, there are also many techniques that help the meditator in her/his efforts; the breath may be a focus, or the teacher may guide the meditators through a guided meditation or steady walking meditation. Mantras, chanting, and singing may be used; specific images or feelings may help to draw the mind of the meditator towards stillness. Meditation teachers and groups are central in this process. Meditation is difficult and can be frustrating. Even the greatest spiritual leaders continue to 'practice'—as, indeed, even the greatest concert pianists also continue to practice. This is a discipline of mind and body that is hard won. Indeed, the calming ways in which meditation relates to mind and body are now supported by neuroscientific research. The functional magnetic resonance imaging scans of experienced and inexperienced meditators taken whilst they are meditating show what meditators have known and experienced for generations: that meditation calms the body, brain, and mind (Davidson et al., 2003; Goleman, 2003: 3–27; Lutz et al., 2004; Ricard, 2007: 186–201).

Naturally, this kind of research encourages the idea of teaching meditation to those who are deeply distressed and who wish to learn, but many of the most needy patients are not able to sit and meditate over a period of time because of the level of their internal agitation and suffering. And whilst clinicians might try to encourage meditation practice, other than in exceptional circumstances, it is unwise to mix the therapeutic role with that of teaching meditation. Meditation should be properly taught by an experienced teacher; therapy should be offered by a well-trained clinician. And even when a clinician is an experienced meditator, it can be confusing other than in moments of crisis, to offer meditation and therapy within the same setting.

However, it is possible that via the psychotherapist's meditative experience, the patient may benefit in different ways. For example, if the meditator is also a psychotherapist who is trying to help traumatized and distressed patients, the meditative practice can enhance the therapist's ability to regulate the patient's anxiety (through affect attunement as described by Stern (1985) and Music (2011: 55–6)) because the capacity to remain calm in the face of the reactive fight–flight anxiety expressed by the patient is enhanced. Gerhardt (2004) describes the evidence about the effects of trauma on the brain as resulting from excessive 'corrosive cortisol' levels. Persistently high levels of cortisol in the brains of babies and young children subjected to severe trauma and abuse literally corrode the brain and body, and form part of a hormonal feedback loop of reactions between brain and body, overstimulating the body's fight–flight responses as a survival mechanism when faced with trauma (Gerhardt, 2004).

With traumatized children who have not had the presence of a caring person to help modulate these responses when they were very young and, indeed, whose carers or parents may have been the source of the trauma, there is a desperate need for the calming presence of another human being if they are to recover their ordinary developmental pathways. The calmness of meditative states of mind within the therapist can be drawn on to make an additional contribution to the calming effect that the therapist needs to have at times on traumatized and reactive patients. This can be a valuable aspect of the 'presence' of the therapist. It is not that the therapist starts to meditate in the session, but that meditative states of mind are an important part of her usual way-of-being. It is part of who the therapist is. The inner calmness can also be absorbed in an unconscious-to-unconscious form of communication where the patient senses this aspect of the therapist's true self and identifies with it in the same way that other aspects of the person of the therapist are identified with, 'unknowingly.' The following clinical example illustrates these possibilities.

Alongside the theoretical and clinical questions raised by of this kind of cross-fertilization and exchange of ideas, there is the need to consider the ways in which new ideas germinate and grow. There is something more solid and thoughtful about a gradual process that develops new ideas; something less 'gimmicky' than many of the technical 'fixes' in which ideas can otherwise be rather too hastily amalgamated. It is my impression that this has been the case with some of the enthusiasm with which mindfulness has been incorporated into evidence-based psychological treatments. Sometimes this enthusiasm has lead to an over-emphasis on the mindfulness technique itself, without understanding the value of the philosophy in which it is rooted. It might be that more can be learnt and gained clinically from the Eastern experiences of meditation than we are as yet aware of as illustrated by the clinical example below.

Playing in the Space Between Meditation and Psychotherapy

One of the great psychoanalytic teachers and thinkers whose ideas are very helpful in developing a dialogue between meditative practice and psychotherapeutic practice is D.W. Winnicott. He did not address these ideas directly: the dialogue between East and West was only coming into being when he died, but his ideas about 'transitional experiences' are fertile ground from which to start. He writes:

> [No] human being is free from the strain of relating inner and outer reality, and relief from this strain is provided by an intermediate area of experience which is not challenged (arts, religion, etc.). This intermediate area is in direct continuity with the play area of the ordinary small child who is 'lost' in play' (1971: 14–15).

Winnicott invites us to think about what is experienced 'in between' that helps to bridge or link very different human experiences. For example, the space/bridge/link between inner and outer reality; the space between two people ('the sphere of between')—the 'I' and 'Thou' that Buber (1985) refers to (Friedman, 1955); the space between the patient and therapist, and how communication takes place between them; the space between a therapy session, home, and school; the space between past and future—which is about 'now', the 'present moment' and 'now-ness'; the dialogue between mindfulness/Buddhism/meditative practice and psychotherapeutic practice.

Winnicott sees this space—sometimes referred to as an intermediate area, other times as a potential space, and other times still as a transitional space—as being full of creative and therapeutic potential for change. The ideas of movement and flow are inherent and are linked with playing which he regards as the developmental bedrock of all human creativity. In this context, what I am trying to do in this chapter is to play with ideas in the space between meditation and psychotherapy.

I have argued elsewhere that the therapist's state of mind during a session is experienced by the patient as the 'presence' of the therapist (Lanyado, 2004). Meditative practice can affect the therapeutic process as a result of the expanded/deepened state of mind of the therapist, of her openness and receptivity to the communications from the patient. The meditative state of mind in the therapist becomes a significant part of her 'presence' when deeply immersed in the therapeutic relationship. Similarly, Winnicott describes as an important phase of ordinary development, when the baby or young child is able to play quietly on his/her own as long as someone important to him/her is emotionally 'present.' He calls this the capacity to be "alone in the presence of someone" (1958: 32).

I would like to draw attention to the ways in which meditative practice enhances the therapist's ability to be emotionally 'present' for the patient, thus enabling the patient to be 'alone' and playing. This wonderfully evocative phrase has several layers of meaning for me. The idea of someone's 'presence' implies authenticity and 'real-ness.' It also implies 'now-ness' and 'being', and, as it extends, it becomes a way of 'dwelling in the present moment', beautifully expressed by the Buddhist teacher Thich Nhat Hanh (2005).

The idea of 'dwelling' resonates with thoughts about holding, staying a while, residing, and is highly relevant to the ways in which the therapist tries to hold the patient in the present moment—an idea, in turn, closely linked to the still and attentive mindfulness of many meditative states.

A Clinical Example of how Meditation Practice can Affect Psychotherapeutic Work

It was my work with Gail that enabled me to see how my meditation practice resonated with my clinical practice. I have written about other aspects of her therapy elsewhere (Lanyado and Horne, 2006; Mortensen and Grunbaum, 2010; Lanyado and Horne, 2012). Grateful to Gail and her family for giving permission for me to write about our work, I will concentrate here on the ways in which I was, I feel, more able to help her because of how meditation helped me.

Gail came for psychotherapy for most of her adolescence. She had been adopted when she was nine years old following neglect, trauma, and abandonment by her vulnerable birth parents. The first few years of her therapy were typical of many children who have had these very unfortunate starts in life. She was highly reactive, unpredictable, and easily angered as a result of a heightened physiological and psychological fight–flight response to all that she had suffered as a young child. She was infuriatingly controlling of the other person in her relationships, and this was understood as a deeply entrenched defence mechanism against her intense anxieties and pain. She couldn't play or talk about her painful feelings of having been rejected and unloved by her birth parents, and tended to express herself through very difficult behavior instead. She would storm out of the therapy room or refuse to come into it. She felt worthless and un-understandable, and that the world was against her.

It was very hard for her to accept the love of her long-suffering adoptive family and she constantly tried their patience and authenticity to the utmost—as, indeed, she did with me in her therapy. During the most chaotic period of her therapy, I think that the fact that I meditated helped me to hang on to a sense of inner calm and stability when with her. The calm inner space created by meditation was like an anchor in the midst of rough seas. I would get tossed around by the waves, but managed to hold on to my therapeutic moorings. In the world outside the consulting room, Gail couldn't concentrate on her schoolwork and was underachieving. Socially she felt, and was, isolated and very different from the other children she met.

Slowly, over the first three years of therapy, Gail became more settled and able to express what she felt, through play and words, rather than action, and I could stop being on high alert in readiness for what on earth she might do next in the sessions. This started with very brief islands of play in the midst of the usual mayhem, and gradually these islands extended into longer periods of time—ten or fifteen minutes at a time. Whilst she was in this state of mind, I could sit and reflect on what she was communicating and she could listen (some of the time) when I tried to put this into words. Mostly, I sat quietly with her, trying to enable her to carry on expressing herself through her play.

Although I had been meditating for many years before her therapy started, my practice had intensified around this time and I think this stillness and open-ness became a stronger part of my way of being with her during the quieter periods in her therapy. This meditative quality, that was becoming an increasingly important part of my way of being, was more openly 'present' in the sessions. Our ways of communicating deepened, allowing the flow of very painful feelings and memories in a way that did not overwhelm Gail with distress.

Thinking in Buber's terms of 'I and Thou', I think we were more able to truly meet during these times and I was very aware of reaching out to her as much as I could through being as available and alert as possible to her smallest communications (Buber, 1985). In psychological language, I became particularly highly attuned to her (Stern, 1985). In psychoanalytic terms, there were more 'moments-of-meeting', which had a strong therapeutic potential to help her to change (ibid).

I also think that the ways in which meditation practice can increase feelings of compassion for and acceptance of difficult feelings and experiences by the meditator, particularly when grounded in a tradition such as Buddhism or Sufism, were important in this process. In my view, it is very difficult to work for many years with people who are suffering in such measure without having developed one's own personal philosophy of what life is about. Whilst meditation practice without these deeper understandings is very helpful in calming the body, mind, and soul, there is very much more to be gained when it is grounded in some understanding of the philosophies and beliefs from which it emerges.

As Gail's narrative of her life was slowly understood through her play, and gradually became more coherent, the beginnings of a mourning process emerged and her life started to make a bit more sense to her. The mourning was first experienced as intense sadness and tearfulness in me before it could be experienced in a bearable way within Gail. She gradually became more able to express her love and gratitude, as well as her anger, towards her adoptive family. She was even able to find some forgiveness towards her birth mother by recognizing her mother's courage in leaving her father to protect herself and her daughter from his violence.

After such a long period of therapy, the ending of our work together was carefully planned and we decided at the start of the school year that she would stop therapy when she went to college. By this time, Gail had spontaneously started to use the couch in her sessions, facing me and reclining on it in an adolescent, chatty kind of way. Here are some notes from one of her last once weekly sessions, where, to my astonishment at the time, a meditative experience took place in the room.

> Gail came into the room and went straight to the couch, re-arranging the cushions to make herself comfortable before lying down. I sat opposite to her in what was my usual chair, which resulted in us facing each other. She said 'What?...' in an aggressive, challenging way—as if feeling persecuted by my looking at her—a familiar theme. I didn't rise to this and just remained quiet. As if to excuse herself for being 'rude' she said: 'I'm just tired' in a stroppy adolescent-ish way. She then chatted inconsequentially about a broken nail, the dark

winter night, how cold it was, and the fact that I had the curtains closed and the lights on. She relaxed on the couch, curling up in a loose foetal position in which I couldn't see her face and then became quiet.

After a while I made a comment which was intended to try to help her to talk if she wished to. She told me that she didn't want to talk and then spent the rest of the session—forty minutes—amazingly still and quiet in this same loose foetal position, but alert and awake. She felt very present and, as had so often been my experience when I had been sitting quietly with her in the past, I felt free to think about and experience the ebb and flow of what this extraordinarily still experience with her could be about.

It felt as if she had entered a quiet, un-persecuted space and I was being allowed to follow her into it, feeling separate but intensely 'present.' The space did not feel sad, depressed or angry. Its strongest quality was its intense stillness. At times it felt as if I was a mother sitting quietly with her baby, not wanting to move in case I disturbed her. But as I became more and more aware of the stillness itself, I was amazed to realise that what I was most aware of was how much the stillness in Gail was like a meditative state.

I found myself thinking of all the different kinds of silence and quietness we had experienced together during her therapy and marvelled at how we had reached this place after all the activity and impulsiveness of the first few years of her therapy. I didn't say any of this to her, not wanting to disrupt the precious state of mind she seemed to be in.

For a while I tried to be as still as she was but realised that I wasn't able to do this despite having meditated in this way for many years. This only served to emphasise to me how extraordinary it was that she was able to stay in this 'place' for as long as she was. As we got closer to the end of the session, I felt that I wanted to say something about what was happening and commented on how different this stillness was from other times we had been quietly together. It seemed to be helping her to feel some peace inside herself. It seemed to be good for her. I realised that what she seemed to be absorbing deeply from me, under the pressure of weekly therapy coming to an end, was that part of me that values these still, meditative states and sees them as being deeply transforming and healing. It was an unconscious identification with a part of me that I had not realised she had somehow perceived.

When I felt that my words would not disrupt the state she was in, I was able to say to her that her ability to reach this stillness was something that would stay with her when she stopped coming to see me each week. It was a place within her, I added, that she could go to when things were hard, that would offer her some peace of mind. It was a link between us and could also be a place of internal refuge to her when she needed it. I didn't refer to the meditative quality of her state of mind as this would have meant little to her. I did draw her attention to it, and describe what she seemed to be experiencing. The session ended, feeling to me like a combination of a therapy session and meditation practice. The sense of stillness remained with her as she left the session.

Whilst I had been very aware of the transformation that had taken place in Gail, it was the contrast between her state of mind in this session and the chaos of her early sessions that stayed with me, and helped me to feel hopeful about her future. During the time of the monthly consultations that followed the end of her weekly therapy, Gail had to face several difficult and distressing life situations. The consultations were very emotional and verbal. It was striking to her parents and to me how sensible, thoughtful, and, indeed, even how wise she became in the face of these difficulties. Could it have been that this was possible because she had become able to use her capacity to sit, be, and dwell with her problems and her distress in a way that enabled her to hold onto a clear sense of direction and values in her young adult life?

Conclusion

Whilst many kinds of cultural activity, such as sports, music, and art, are very helpful in calming and focusing the mind and body in the present moment, meditation practice does this directly, using time-honored techniques to calm and still the mind in ways that can become part of the true self of the therapist. This can become advantageous to patients, particularly when the therapist becomes able to dwell in the present moment for longer periods of time.

This raises the intriguing question of whether experiencing the present moment intensely might have the power to counteract intense experiences from the past so the past experiences no longer get confused with what is happening now. Separating past and present can be a central therapeutic challenge for traumatized patients. Enabling them to experience the reality of time—that was then, this is now—can be a major therapeutic breakthrough. By learning through meditative practice to be very much in the present, the therapist may be able to create a therapeutic space in which the present moment is fully experienced and the past is truly left where it belongs.

References

Black, D.M. (ed.) (2006) *Psychoanalysis and Religion in the 21st Century: Competitors or Collaborators?* (London: Routledge).

Black, D.M. (2011) *Why Things Matter: The Place of Values in Science, Psychoanalysis and Religion* (London/New York: Routledge).

Buber, M. (1985) *Between Man and Man*, translated by Ronald Gregor Smith (London/New York: Routledge).

Coltart, N. (1992) *Slouching Towards Bethlehem . . . And Further Psychoanalytic Explanations* (New York: Guilford Press).

Coltart, N. (1993) *How to Survive as a Psychotherapist* (London: Sheldon Press).

Coltart, N. (ed.) (1996) *The Baby and the Bathwater* (London: Karnac).

Concise Oxford English Dictionary of Current English (1990) (Oxford: Clarendon Press).

Davidson, R.J., Kabat-Zinn, J., Schumacher, J., Rosenkranz, M., Muller, D., Santorelli, S. F., et al. (2003) 'Alterations in Brain and Immune Function Produced by Mindfulness Meditation', *Psychosomatic Medicine*, 65, 564–70.

Eigen, M. (2008) 'Primary Aloneness', *Psychoanalytic Perspectives*, 5(2), 63–8.

Epstein, M. (1995) *Thoughts Without a Thinker* (New York: Basic Books).

Epstein, M. (2006) 'The Structure of no Structure: Winnicott's Concept of Unintegration and the Buddhist Notion of No-self', in Black, D. M. (ed.) *Psychoanalysis and Religion in the 21st Century. Competitors or Collaborators?*, pp. 223–33 (London: Routledge).

Freud, S. (1939) *Moses and Monotheism* (London: Hogarth Press and Institute of Psycho-Analysis).

Friedman, M. (1955) *Martin Buber: The Life of Dialogue*, 4th edition (2002) (London: Routledge).

Gerhardt, S. (2004) *Why Love Matters* (Hove: Routledge).

Goleman, D. (2003) *Destructive Emotions and How We Can Overcome Them: A Dialogue with The Dalai Lama Narrated by Daniel Goleman* (London: Bloomsbury).

Hanh, T.N. (2005) *Being Peace* (Berkeley, CA: Parallax Press).

Kabat-Zinn, J. (1990) *Full Catastrophe Living. How to Cope with Stress, Pain and Illness Using Mindfulness Meditation* (London: Piatkus Books).

Lanyado, M. (2004) *The Presence of the Therapist* (Hove: Brunner-Routledge).

Lanyado, M. and Horne, A. (eds) (2006) *A Question of Technique* (Hove: Routledge).

Lanyado, M. and Horne, A. (eds) (2012) *Winnicott's Children: Independent Psychoanalytic Approaches with Children and Adolescents* (London/New York: Routledge).

Lutz, A., Greischar, L.L., Rawlings, N.B., Ricard, M. and Davidson, R.J. (2004) 'Long-term Meditators Self-induce High Amplitude Gamma Synchrony During Mental Practice', *Proceedings of the National Academy of Sciences of the United States of America*, 101, 46.

McGilchrist, I. (2009) *The Master and his Emissary: The Divided Brain and the Making of the Western World* (New Haven, CT: Yale University Press).

Molino, A. (ed.) (1998) *The Couch and the Tree: Dialogues in Psychoanalysis and Buddhism* (New York: North Point Press).

Mortensen, K. V. and Grunbaum, L. (eds) (2010) *Play and Power*, European Federation of Psychoanalytic Psychotherapists (EFPP) Book Series (London: Karnac Books).

Music, G. (2011) *Nurturing Natures. Attachment and Children's Emotional, Sociocultural and Brain Development* (Hove: Psychology Press).

Parsons, M. (ed.) (2000) *The Dove That Returns, the Dove That Vanishes* (London: Routledge).

Parsons, M. (2006) 'Ways of Transformation', in Black, D. M. (ed.) *Psychoanalysis and Religion in the 21st Century: Competitors or Collaborators?*, pp. 117–31 (London: Routledge).

Ricard, M. (2007) *Happiness* (London: Atlantic Books).

Rubin, J.B. (2006) 'Psychoanalysis and Spirituality', in Black, D. M. (ed.) *Psychoanalysis and Religion in the 21st Century: Competitors or Collaborators?*, pp. 132–53 (London: Routledge).

Segal, Z. V., Williams, J, M. G. and Teasdale, J. D. (2002) *Mindfulness-based Cognitive Therapy for Depression: A New Approach to Preventing Relapse* (New York: Guildford Press).

Stern, D. (1985) *The Interpersonal World of the Infant* (New York: Basic Books).

Symington, N. (1994) *Emotion and Spirit: questioning the Claims of Psychoanalysis and Religion* (London: Continuum).

Winnicott, D.W. (ed.) (1958) *The Maturational Processes and the Facilitating Environment* (London: Hogarth Press).

Winnicott, D.W. (1971) *Playing and Reality* (London: Tavistock; reprinted 1974 Harmondsworth: Pelican).

Concluding Unmindful Postscript

The mindfulness phenomenon that has swept the mental health field for the last two decades has been unashamedly *secular* in style and substance—admirably so. It has helped dispel some of Buddhism's holy mist—often a screen for unholy and (as with most religions) power-driven shenanigans.

It would be naïve, however, to think that our instinctive human longing for the sacred can be satisfied by a diet of weekly exercises, cognitive rewiring, behavioural reprogramming, and regular self-congratulatory forays into the working of our neurons.

It would be equally naïve to delegate self-appointed 'trans-personal' and 'spiritual' practitioners and 'guides' with the task of providing us with a foldable pocket size map of our own path. This is because we *create* a path as we walk (and often stumble) on uncertain and uncharted terrain.

From Kierkegaard—author of *Concluding Unscientific Postscript* (1992), hence a tutelary presence in these retrospective musings—one learns how in turn exciting, despairing, and even dangerous a genuine search for the sacred truly is, and how remote from the self-satisfied imperturbability often associated with mindfulness and Buddhism.

The *emergence* of the sacred always catches us unawares; it materialises in the phenomenal world (where else?) when we least expect it, unless, of course, we truly believe that this dimension can be manufactured. If this were the case, then experience would simply be an offshoot of the self rather than belonging to a more expansive domain.

The emergence of the sacred need not be transcendental or other-worldly. It is often *evoked*; it often appears *in disguise*. One has to be able to read between the lines, in what is being suggested by notions such as the actualising tendency, the unconscious communication between client and therapist, infinite resonance, emptiness, symmetrical thought, I–Thou, the organism and organismic experiencing, mindfulness, nirvana... the list could go on. When not *reified*—that is, turned into solid *things*, but allowed to remain fluid pointers—these various notions indicate a richer area of exploration than the one envisaged by a necessarily limited self and by the conscious mind.

Recoiling from the literalism of *McMindfulness* as a quick fix for the anxieties of late-capitalist society, a more nuanced interpretation of meditation would make a practitioner more open to its deeper meaning.

Mindfulness—in the diverse and creative interpretations found in this book—could then be understood as the cultivation of a sensibility receptive to the emergence of the sacred in the mundane. Personally, I see the sacred as what escapes purpose—a dimension not unlike play. How one *describes* the sacred—or, indeed, what term one chooses in its place—will, of course, vary. What is less easily disputable is that it occurs within the world of phenomena, in the *Lebenswelt*, in our lived life—in that very dimension that many religious traditions (including Buddhism) chose to despise and denigrate.

Long before sending invitations out to contributors, I had envisioned this collection as an example of *dependent-arising*, the Buddha's original notion often interpreted (more or less correctly) as 'inter-dependence.' To a certain degree, this is what took place here: each of the perspectives developed in the book is tacitly impacted (when not directly informed) by different, at times even opposing, views—adding, perhaps, a refreshingly *dialectical* spin to the Buddha's insight.

Some readers would have found it preferable, I assume, to come across a cluster of views joined in mutual and uncontroversial dialogue. These imaginary readers may have preferred to read yet another book on mindfulness in step with a notion of pluralism in vogue at present. In the name of universalism, this view effectively promotes homogenisation, that is, bland sameness. Whereas universalism looks for the common ground yet seemingly respecting cultural and anthropological specificities, its cruder implementation results in homogenisation, that is, the bending of specificities to the appetites of a pre-existing agenda.

Genuine dialogue is, of course, paramount, in the same way as an 'integrative' and even 'integral' search for common ground is, in theory, able to foster communication among practitioners, thinkers, and researchers. But we simply cannot afford to bypass the cultural and historical specificities of every single approach to meditation and/or psychology. That would be a disservice to their richness and uniqueness. Yet this is what is arguably taking place at present in most 'integrative' psychotherapy and counselling courses, as well as in 'non-denominational' meditation retreats and mindfulness programmes.

There is something disingenuous in arbitrarily mixing Freud and Rogers with a sprinkle of Maslow and a dash of Bowlby. There is something gratuitous in blending Zen with Tibetan Buddhism, adding an incongruous touch of Christian mysticism and New Age shamanism. In doing so, we miss out on the inimitability and sheer otherness of the particular. We also end up serving a misguided 'universalist' agenda that bends every cultural, religious, and psychological manifestation to the needs of the market.

What struck me, after repeated reading, is how neatly the highly diverse essays offered here portray—even within the necessary limited confines of a conversation on meditation and psychology—our post-metaphysical condition. 'Post-metaphysical' is a rather grand way of saying that in spite of our ever-present need for certainties the days of metaphysics are over.

Already two centuries ago, Nietzsche heralded its demise in his jabs at the Platonic tradition. He referred to metaphysics as *Hinterwelt*, 'the back world', a doctrine assuming the existence of a world *behind* the curtain of appearance. He similarly poked fun at *Hinterweltler*, back-world-persons (Adorno, 2001), people like Luther who had squandered their genuine talent for the philosophical life and the art of living only to get embroiled in back-world pursuits such as religion and theology.

A post-metaphysical world is, by definition, *perspectival*: it takes for granted that every claim to ultimate (or even relative) truth is yet another perspective, and it cannot announce itself as the God's eye view without being laughed at. To this I would add that a *critical*, philosophically-engaged practice would be equally alert to the substantial differences between *multiplicity* and *pluralism*. The former implies openness to honest disagreement and even rupture in the service of the greater good. The latter, all the rage in contemporary political discourse, favours compromise in the name of peaceful co-existing and often amounts to little more than shallow eclecticism, to picking and choosing from the shelves of the *perennial wisdom supermarket*.

The contemporary metropolis embodies, for some, the essence of multiplicity. It is a *chaosmos*—chaos *and* cosmos, a tuneful pandemonium with each living voice modulating its hum in the wake of a neighbouring sound.

Lyotard (1984) asked whether all the different cultures living side by side in a big city are really talking and listening to one another. In his film, *Code Inconnu*, the Austrian director Michael Haneke (2000) makes a similar point. They both seem to imply that genuine dialogue, if and when it happens, is an *accident* and simply cannot be manufactured beforehand by any agenda. This, perhaps, grants it a higher degree of legitimacy than one that is motivated by a utilitarian need for mere co-existence.

Lyotard and Haneke also seem to imply that in our contemporary world different cultures and traditions often live parallel lives, that is, they co-exist without really talking to or being impacted by one another. This has been my own experience over many years as an active member of Buddhist and Western therapeutic communities and associations. A distinctive *campanilismo* (the bell tower syndrome, according to which the bell tower in *my* hometown has a crisper and more cheerful sound than yours) mars effective exploration favouring, instead, parochial leanings. Whether characterised by claims of authenticity or greater depth, of a more direct link to the historical Buddha or special probity, of greater commitment to the client or deeper understanding of the patient's unconscious, these explicit and implicit statements all aim to inflate the importance of one's own tribe and parish.

Not being impacted by the other means to forfeit the very possibility of learning, if one believes, as I do, that education is not Platonic *maieutics* (bringing forth, with the help of a 'midwife' what is already latent in one) but impact with otherness (Levinas, 1961), with what is external to one's tribe and nation.

In spite of the multiplicity of views offered, the reader may agree that a common ethos transpires in these writings. They all seem to point to the fact that, after nearly three decades of 'mindfulness', it is now high time to benefit from the lessons learned, acknowledge the contribution offered by the mindfulness programmes, and bring the level of practice, theory, and research in the field of meditation and psychology to a deeper level. Setting this ambitious project in motion also describes the aspiration behind this book.

The future is uncertain, and maybe this is a good thing. The Buddha's teachings offer a great reservoir of wisdom and compassion, and none of us really know how they will be absorbed and integrated in years to come. Commenting on Kierkegaard, Jacques Derrida (2007) wrote that Christianity is still to come. Might the same be true of Buddhism? One of my students was annoyed by the suggestion. She objected that Christianity was present each time an individual embodied its message of love and forgiveness. Could something similar be true of mindfulness and of the Dharma? Would it be enough for an individual to fully embrace the Buddha's teaching for the Dharma to be actualised? Or would a more encompassing, civic vision be necessary?

There are times, in clinical work as in life, when we do need certainty, and more or less fathom our next step. At other times, it may be good to wonder whether that very same attitude is ruled by fear. We would then opt for *not* having a pre-conceived idea and be prepared, instead, to respond to what comes up.

As a client told me recently, "There are times when I *don't* want to know what's around the corner."

Manu Bazzano
August 2013

References

Adorno, T. (2001) *Metaphysics: Concept and Problems* (Cambridge: Polity).
Derrida, J. (2007) *The Gift of Death* (Chicago, IL: Chicago University Press).
Haneke, M. (2000) *Code Unknown: Incomplete Tales of Several Journeys*, a film by Michael Haneke, produced by Marin Karmitz.
Kierkegaard, S. (1992) *Concluding Unscientific Postscript to Philosophical Fragments*, vol. 1 (Princeton, NJ: Princeton University Press).
Levinas, E. (1961) *Totality and Infinity: An Essay on Exteriority* (Pittsburgh, PA: Duquesne University Press).
Lyotard, J. F. (1984) *The Postmodern Condition: A Report on Knowledge* (Minneapolis, MN: University of Minnesota).

Index

non-dualistic approach, 81, 91,
97, 98
non-evident v. evident, in human
experience, 113, 117, 119

objects, 29, 127, 131–2
obsessive compulsive disorder, 139
Olson, C., 131, 133
other-centered paradigm, 23–36, 46

pain, 91, 118
Pāli Canon, 26, 43, 101
panic disorder, 139–40
Panksepp, J., 73
Panopticon, 88–90
paraphilia, 93
Parsons, M., 149, 150
Payge, Mark, 61, 62
Perls, F. S., 141
phenomenology, 68, 114, 127, 131
embodied, 32–4
philosophical assessment, of
mindfulness, 49–60
physics, 103
Pilgrim, D., 83
play, 51, 155–6
pluralism, 164, 165
Popper, K., 15
positivist psychology, 61, 63,
71, 89
post-metaphysical world, 165
post-modernity, 53, 101–3,
107, 110
Prakriti, 145
presence, 155, 156
present moment
awareness, 24, 25, 33, 119, 137
here and now, 54
practice, 104, 107, 108
in psychotherapy, 156, 160, 161
recollection, 6, 11
problem-solving mindfulness,
105, 106
programming
human genetic, 141
levels of, 141
local cultural, 141
perinatal, 141
personal historical, 141

prehistoric, 141
selves and, 140–1
protective awareness, 8–9, 19
Protestantism, 68, 75
Proust, M., 71
psychoanalytical psychotherapy,
148–62
psychotherapist, *see* therapist
psychotherapy
clinical examples, 64–6, 156–60
clinical mindfulness, 136–47
goal-setting, 141–2
meditation and, 148–62
Panopticon and, 89
paths of therapeutic change,
136–7
programs, 140–1
psychoanalytical, 148–62
skeptical approach, 112–23
Purser, R., 75–6
Pyrrho, 112–13, 114, 118–19
Pyrrhonian skepticism, 112–19

quadrilemma, 117

Rāmāyaṇa, 5–6
rationalism, 53
recollection, 5–6, 43–4
Relate, 94
relationship therapy, 81–100
relaxation techniques, 52
religion, 16–17, 63, 75, 164, 165
religious Buddhism, 3, 14–15, 16–17,
68, 70
remembrance, 57, 138
bad life, 70
mindfulness as, 24–6, 30
of sacred, 30, 33
of texts, 5–6
resentment, 63
reverie, 71–2
Rhys Davids, T. W., 49, 56
Ricard, M., 153
Richards, C., 94
Right Mindfulness (*sammā sati*), 11
Rogers, C., 59
romantic relationships, 94–7, 98
Rorty, R., 124
Rose, H., 72

174   *Index*

therapist, 33–4
  interpersonal start to therapy, 137
  meditative states, 148–62
  presence of, 156
therapy, 57, 63
  therapeutic spirituality, 34–5
  see also psychotherapy
thoughts, 104–5, 106, 107–8,
    136–7, 138
three bodies of Buddha, 143–4
thusness, 62, 71–2, 73
Tolstoy's question, 104, 110
tonglen practice, 96
toothpaste-tube therapy, 136
traditional authority, 102–3, 104
Transactional Analysis, 141
transitional experiences, 155
trauma
  in childhood and adolescence, 149,
    154, 156–61
  fight–flight responses, 154,
    156–7
treatment, mindfulness not, 57–8
true nature, 141–3, 144–5
Turnbull, D., 141

unconscious, 72, 115
  distraction and, 54–6
  revisited, 73–4

vaginismus, 91
Varela, F. J., 90
vedana (reaction), 26, 28, 31–2
Vendler, H., 76

vipassanā tradition, 12, 13, 18,
    106, 143
Virgil, 69

walking mindfully, 63
Wallis, G., 6, 16
Walser, R. D., 95
Wang, Y., 124
washing teacup mindfully, 25–6
Watts, A., 126
Weber, M., 104
Wellwood, J., 96, 97
Western mindfulness, 84–6, 87–8
Western scientific model, of
    cause–effect relationships, 83, 90
Western therapeutic approaches, to
    suffering, 83–4
Western world, and post-modernity,
    101–11
Westrup, D., 95
Williams, J. M. G., 82
Williams, M., 18, 19, 138
Williams, P., 143
Winnicott, D. W., 155, 156
Wittgenstein, L., 37, 124

Young, J. E., 141

Zen
  koan, 59
  shoji, 61
  practice, 83
  zazen, 88
Zen vow, 40
Zupancic, A., 66

Printed and bound by CPI Group (UK) Ltd, Croydon, CR0 4YY